THE DRY CHALLENGE

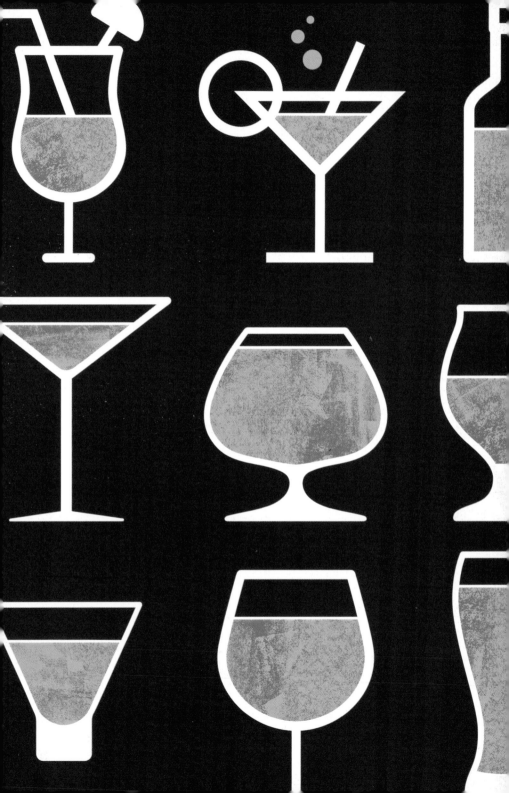

THE DRY CHALLENGE

HOW TO LOSE THE BOOZE FOR DRY JANUARY, SOBER OCTOBER, AND ANY OTHER ALCOHOL-FREE MONTH

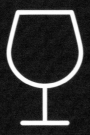

HILARY SHEINBAUM
FOREWORD BY LO BOSWORTH

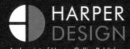

HARPER DESIGN
An Imprint of HarperCollins Publishers

HarperCollins books may be purchased for educational, business, or sales promotional use. For information please email the Special Markets Department at SPsales@harpercollins.com.

First published in 2020 by
Harper Design
An Imprint of HarperCollinsPublishers
195 Broadway
New York, NY 10007
Tel: (212) 207-7000
Fax: (855) 746-6023
harperdesign@harpercollins.com
www.hc.com

Distributed by
HarperCollinsPublishers
195 Broadway
New York, NY 10007

ISBN 978-0-06-293770-4
Library of Congress Control Number: 2020017946

Printed in the United States of America

Second Printing, 2020

For Alejandro

Thanks for making a bet . . .
keeping your side of the wager,
and, uh . . . being a great friend.

Contents

Foreword

In 2015, I was not really myself. I was off, dizzy, anxious, and just not well. I am someone who has always strived to live a healthy lifestyle, but that seemed to have been lost in that period of my life. I saw doctor after doctor until we eventually found the source—a severe vitamin deficiency. After finding the root cause of my issues, I was able to begin a healing journey that would ultimately lead me even deeper into my mission for wellness.

Now, you might be wondering, what does any of that have to do with Dry January? Two things: I am a New Yorker, having lived in the city for more than ten years, and I have an extensive culinary background. So what do these two things have in common? Alcohol. Yes, alcohol. In our society, especially in busy, bustling metropolitan areas, it is quite common for alcohol to be at the center of all social activity. This is something that I am not a stranger to. Alcohol is at the center of both the New York social scene and the culinary industry. It's just there, and it almost feels expected that you participate, even if it's *just one* perfect cocktail at a Michelin-star restaurant in Greenwich Village.

As someone who was trying to heal herself internally and become well again, it seemed like the perfect opportunity to participate in Dry January. I heard about the challenge from a friend and was motivated by the potential of what it could do for my body and mind. I decided to take it on and see how my healing journey would be affected and how it might change my social interactions.

I don't want you to get the impression I'm a big drinker, by any means; I just enjoy a nice tequila on the rocks at dinner with friends. Having a drink felt like the thing to do, so when I took on this challenge, there was a shift. It was, well, strange. It felt odd to not order a glass of wine or say, "Let's go for drinks!" after a long day at work. While my challenge and decision got a few initial questions from friends, most were supportive. It became somewhat liberating not to depend on drinking for socializing. In addition to feeling liberated, it helped me feel like I was supporting the actions I had already implemented to heal my body. My skin was clear and I had more energy than I had had in a long time. I was able to sleep better and think clearer. The Dry January challenge turned into another tool in my arsenal for healing.

My friend Hilary Sheinbaum captures the ins and outs of Dry January perfectly in this book. I've known Hilary to be a writer, journalist, wellness enthusiast, and an overall realist. This book is the most relatable how-to–meets–memoir I've read yet. She outlines a step-by-step guide to conquering a Dry January all while offering her own experiences—which can help with any Dry Challenge. She answers every question you could possibly have about its before, during, and aftereffects and gives you an inside look to her own challenges with a dry month. This book doesn't just help answer all of your questions—you also feel as if you've found a friend in Hilary with whom you can go through a possibly challenging month (especially if none of your real-life friends is willing to give up their glass of Pinot Noir!).

Lo Bosworth, *founder and CEO of Love Wellness*

Hi and Dry AF

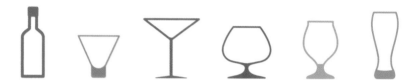

I was first introduced to the idea of Dry January—the self-imposed pact to abstain from all forms of alcohol for the entire month—by one of my friends, Alejandro (aka Al). The first time we met was at a pre-party get-together in my New York City apartment during the winter of 2014. He was a guest of a guest, and brought a bottle of vodka for the occasion as a hostess gift (thanks, bud). Fast-forward to December 2016, during the month of boozy holiday get-togethers and birthdays, work-induced drinking activities, and an excessive number of unnecessary late nights, when Al and I had a casual dinner to hang out and catch up. Over sushi, he told me about a friend who had pledged to not drink during the following month. I almost fell out of my seat. I'm pretty sure I paused with my nigiri mid-chopstick-lift and responded with a dropped jaw.

"Why?"

Al explained: The previous year, his friend had given up all forms of booze—wine, beer, and spirits—for one whole month (bravo to you, I thought). This guy had successfully completed the challenge and wouldn't shut up about how amazing he had felt during and after his drink-free January. The friend was going to attempt it again. Al was considering it, too. "Interesting," I noted to myself. It was definitely a thought-provoking take on a typical New Year's resolution. At this stage in my career, I had been writing about a variety of topics, but I was mostly covering food and beverage: everything from chefs, restaurants, mixologists, and bars to wine and, of course, cocktails. I didn't consider myself an excessive drinker, then—maybe two drinks a night twice each week—or even now, but my job certainly presented a number of opportunities, for, um, tastings and fun times with alcoholic beverages. (I believe the technical term is "first-hand research.")

Almost immediately following the next few bites of sashimi and salmon rolls, I totally forgot about Dry January (truthfully, sushi has that shiny-object-attention-grabbing effect on me, like a Golden Retriever spotting a tennis ball . . . no offense, Dry Jan!). But, one week after Al enlightened me, on New Year's Eve 2016, with a glass of Champagne in my hand (with no tasty tuna on the table to distract me) and no prospects for a New Year's goal, I remembered my friend's intention to eliminate alcohol from his agenda. And so, before the ball-drop countdown began, over text message, we decided to make a bet. The premise? Who could stay sober for thirty-one days straight. The person who had one drink (even one silly sip of a beer)—ahem, the "loser"—would treat the winner to dinner at any restaurant in New York City. (The list included Michelin-starred venues Eleven Madison Park, Per Se, and Momofuku Ko.) If we both won Dry January, we'd split the bill. If we both failed, there would be no feasting on fancy food for these friends who failed to remain dry. "Happy New Year!" I wished my friend as midnight struck.

And just like that, we had a bet. And thirty-one days to go.

That first year of Dry January was definitely the most challenging for me. For one, I went in completely unprepared. It was something I decided to do on a whim (more specifically: less than five minutes before 2017 while consuming an unusual amount of bubbly. It was, after all, New Year's Eve). I learned everything I know about Dry January by doing it—yes, by simply participating. Sure, I listened to advice (both helpful and not-so-great ideas), but at the time there were few people (at least within my immediate social circles) who were participating in this cultural phenomenon. Some of my friends were skeptical. Others were supportive. Many rolled their eyes in disbelief (or frustration, or just indifference). But I had Al to back me up. He was my Sober Month Support Squad (party of two), right? Well . . . for a minute anyway.

Long story short: Al lost. I won a very nice supper paid for by my dear friend, thanks to my stubbornness in remaining dry and his inability to pass up a beer (under peer pressure).

In the end, I won a lot more than I bargained for.

Don't get me wrong, the tasting menu at Momofuku Ko is phenomenal (thanks again, friend!), but this bet impacted my days, my overall month, and my perspective about much more than drinking. It also changed my thoughts about alcohol (and forgoing booze . . . well, sometimes) for the rest of 2017, and beyond. It truly altered my routine, for the better.

Years later (fast-forward to the present day), Al will never make a bet with me about anything ever again. With that said, despite not having a tasty meal motivating me to reach the finish line, I still participate in this thirty-one-day resolution every year from January 1 to February 1.

That's how it started for me.

Dry January: Party Like It's Prohibition

January. It's the longest month of the year. Okay, there are other months with thirty-one days, but January *feels* like the longest. You've just spent the previous six-ish weeks stuffing turkeys and yourself, trimming trees and downing eggnog, and hopping from holiday party to holiday party, having a glass or two (or four) of the festive cocktail being served. Or maybe you hunkered down in the increasingly chilly weather, polishing off bottles of wine and binge-watching your favorite TV series.

Maybe you were lucky and took an actual vacation during the holiday season: somewhere warm and beachy, where you sipped tropical drinks with little umbrellas and fresh fruit garnishes, or somewhere alpine where you gathered around the fire for warming après-ski beverages. However you ended your year, there were likely many drinks involved. (No judgment.) And now, here you are, on the doorstep of January, feeling overfed, overserved, and so over feeling hungover. You want to start the new year off right. You want to reset. Detox. Go dry.

Dry January, "Dry Jan," "Dryuary," or "Dryanuary" is the act of giving up all forms of alcohol—wine, beer, spirits, and cocktails for thirty-one days—the entire first month of the year. That means: no shots, no low-ABV cocktails, and no Champagne toasts (although you can cheers without sipping if it suits you!).

While this goal may sound intimidating or even scary, rest assured: It's a far cry from a mandatory prohibition. Dry January is not a life sentence, a financial commitment, or an undertaking you have to take on alone (or in secret, for that matter). In fact, tons of people partake in no-drinking Januarys across the globe.

Outside of a drink-free January, people of all ages have flirted with—or at least become interested in—the idea of abstaining from alcohol for periods of time longer than thirty-one days. Participating in this highly publicized movement is a great way to test those waters for long-term commitment.

> PRO TIP: **IF YOU'RE YEARNING FOR A COMPLETELY SOBER LIFESTYLE YEAR-ROUND (AND BEYOND) BUT FEEL INTIMIDATED BY THE UNDERTAKING, START WITH DRY JANUARY AND SEE WHERE IT LEADS YOU!**

Beginnings: From Across the Bar—er—Pond

The term "Dry January" was coined in the UK.

1984 **Campaigning nonprofit Alcohol Concern** (now Alcohol Change UK) was founded with the goal of reducing the harm that can be caused by alcohol.

2011 **Dry January's story began** with a woman living in the UK named Emily Robinson, who signed up for her first half marathon. In preparation for the long run, she decided to cut out alcohol—specifically, during her January training, creating a dry month. Her experiment was a success! She reported losing weight, feeling increased energy, and sleeping better.

2012 **Because her experience yielded beneficial results,** Emily decided to forgo booze in January, again. That same month, she started a new job, as the chief deputy executive at Alcohol Concern.

Once she became part of the Alcohol Concern team, people (not just Emily) were talking about the positive changes that occur when one cuts out beer, wine, and spirits for the entire month, following all the holiday boozing. It got the charity's team thinking: If it could get more people to take a break from drinking in January, would more people think about their drinking habits? And would they consume fewer boozy beverages after those thirty-one days were over? The team also wondered if they could promote this idea to a larger audience and inspire people to engage in conversations that highlight the great things that happen when you take a break from drinking. (Spoiler alert: All these hypotheticals became realities.)

2013 **The first official Dry January** took place in the UK, with about four thousand participants who signed up for supportive emails via the Alcohol Concern website.

During the first Dry January campaign, UK journalist and political aide Alastair Campbell discussed his past—in relation to booze—and columnist Peter Osborne wrote about his first-person experience partaking in the month-long challenge. Simultaneously, that inaugural year, people in the UK were (pleasantly) arguing: Are there long-term changes that stem from giving up alcohol for one month? Meanwhile Dr. Richard de Visser from the University of Sussex volunteered to survey participants and see what effects it had on them. The doc had big news! He found that six months after Dry Jan, almost seven out of ten people continued to consume fewer quantities of booze than before!

2014 **Midyear,** the charity trademarked "Dry January."

2015 **In January,** Public Health England, an executive agency of the Department of Health and Social Care in the UK, funded promotion in support of this month-long commitment to sobriety (but only for a year, and now Dry January is completely independent of government support).

2017 **In April,** the charity merged with another organization, Alcohol Research UK, and renamed itself Alcohol Change UK. The new shared identity was announced in November 2018.

A lot of stuff happened in between and after, but you get the gist! Things were moving forward. People were taking notice. And not only were they paying attention, they were deciding not to drink for (you guessed it!) an entire month.

Shout out to Finland! In 1942, decades before Emily Robinson laced up her running shoes, Finland started the program Raitis Tammikuu (in English, "Sober January") to aid the war effort against the Soviet Union.

Thanks to these two trendy European trailblazing countries, Dry January has become a global phenomenon, with millions participating (and more and more) each year.

. . . Now, It's Your Turn

Why would *you* do such a thing during the (seemingly) longest, darkest, coldest month of the year?

Beyond solidifying a New Year's resolution, perhaps you want to explore a new you in the new year. If you slacked off at the office in December, Dry January may be a good time to dig into work without distraction and save hard-earned cash. Some unexpected benefits might come of this, too (like clearer, healthier-looking skin). You might start a trend in your friend circle (and meet new people) and also realize the best ways to spend your free time! The perks to taking on this challenge are endless.

Now Dry January is so popular that other months are competing, with their own no-booze challenges. Dry Feb/Sober February, Dry July, Sober September, Sober October, and No-Alcohol November/ No-Drink November are a few. Note that the lessons learned during Dry January (and from reading this book) can apply to any month-long period. February is a few days shorter than January. September has one fewer twenty-four-hour period than January does. And although October has the same number of days, it doesn't feel as long as the first month of the year. Each month has its own challenges, for sure, but the outcome is the same: a commitment to no alcohol for an extended period of time. (Also, you're not confined to begin on the first day of the month—any start date will do!)

In this book you'll find everything you need to know about how to complete Dry January (or Sober October, or any other alcohol-free month). It'll cover how to prepare for the booze-free weeks ahead, how to let friends and family know about your undertaking (and how to respond when someone tries to sabotage it!), and what to do if you slip up and have a drink (or two) before your challenge concludes. Included are ideas for fun nonboozy activities, recipes for nonalcoholic or "zero-proof" drinks (two terms commonly preferred over "mocktails"), and how to commemorate reaching February 1 (or November 1, or the end of whatever month you choose).

Pour yourself a tall, cold glass of sparkling water and let's get started!

Dry **January**
Dry **February**
Sober **March**
Alcohol-Free **April**
Mocktail **May**
Dry **June**
Dry **July**
Alcohol-Free **August**
Sober **September**
Sober **October**
No-Drink **November**
Dry **December**

By-the-Glass

This isn't your typical glossary. Truth be told: these definitions aren't fact-checked by any governing language authority or standards other than . . . this book. Pinky-swear promise: There is no pop quiz at the end of this glossary. Glance over these fun words, or take a deep dive. The choice is yours! If you need to reference any terms as you read through the upcoming chapters, bounce back here to freshen up. There's even room to add your own quirky expressions, as you see fit.

ALCOHOL the substance you will not be drinking during a sober month

BAR a place that serves alcohol, where you may spend less time during your dry challenge

BEER a beverage you will not be drinking during your month-long hiatus from booze (unless it is nonalcoholic)

BOOZE another word for alcohol

COCKTAILS alcoholic beverages with one or more spirits mixed, stirred, or shaken with ingredients like juice, syrup, or other elements . . . which you will not be drinking during a dry month

DAMP JANUARY a less boozy month (in comparison with the months that precede it)

DEMI-SEC a reference to medium-dry wine, which can also be applied to a medium-dry month

DRINKING the act of sipping, gulping, and ultimately consuming liquid (likely alcohol)

DRYATHALON the seemingly marathon-length twenty-eight to thirty-one days when persons forgo all wine, beer, and spirits (most commonly during January)

DRY FEBRUARY the act of giving up all alcohol (wine, beer, spirits) for twenty-eight days of the month; it can be an alternative to, a consolation to not finishing, or a continuation of Dry January

DRY JANUARY the act of giving up all alcohol (wine, beer, spirits) for thirty-one days of the month; also known as Dryuary, Dry Jan, Dryanuary, Dryathalon. The term was coined in the UK and trademarked in 2014 by the charity Alcohol Concern (which is now known as Alcohol Change UK after merging with Alcohol Research UK)

DRY JULY thirty-one days of summery weather, which may involve swimsuits, sunscreen, and celebrating America's independence with fireworks. Does not include: refreshing ice-cold cocktails, any type of alcoholic spritz, or frosty beers

FEBRUARY a time when you can drink again (if you want to/if you are not participating in Dry February)!

"HAPPY NEW YEAR!" the first words of the new year, and your signal to start Dry January. Put the drink down—it's go time!

HANGOVER/HUNGOVER an uncomfortable, unfortunate, and inevitable feeling of nausea and/or head pounding, spell of dehydration and/or tummy problems caused by drinking too much. You will not experience (or miss this) during January, or any other sober month

MOCKTAILS like cocktails, but without the alcoholic component

N.A. BEVERAGES "Non" + "Alcoholic," meaning drinks that do not contain—you guessed it—alcohol

NO-DRINK NOVEMBER refraining from consuming all alcoholic beverages during the thirty days leading up to December (. . . in anticipation of holiday parties the following month, or to allot extra calories for Thanksgiving dinner)!

ONE-DRINK JANUARY when a completely booze-free Dry January is the goal, but a big (or small occasion) permits one drink (or one night of drinking) during the month

SOBER the act of not consuming alcohol; not drinking

SOBER FEBRUARY see Dry February

SOBER OCTOBER the act of giving up all alcohol (wine, beer, spirits) for thirty-one days of the month: sometimes it's an alternative to or consolation for not finishing Dry January

SOBER SEPTEMBER fresh off summer vacation (filled with sugary, sippable drinks), this is another month you can give up alcohol for thirty days; a post-summer detox, if you will

SOBER MONTH SUPPORT SQUAD one person or a group of cheerleaders who fully supports the commitment to Dry January and other dry months. Can be friends, coworkers, family members, or even acquaintances who are also participating in the Dryathlon

SPIRITS hard alcohol (i.e., vodka, tequila, whiskey); in short: liquids you will not be drinking

THIRTY-ONE DAYS the number of twenty-four-hour periods in January (as well as some other months); it is also the amount of time you will refrain from consuming boozy beverages

WINE made of grapes. Can be red, rosé, orange, white, sparkling, whatever you choose. Also, a beverage you will not be drinking during your sober month (unless it's nonalcoholic)

In Your Own Words

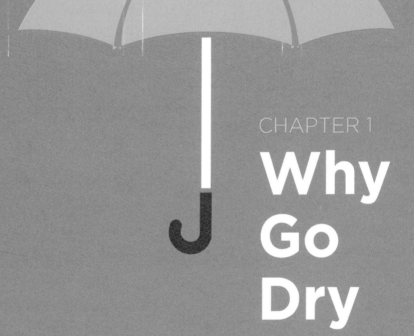

CHAPTER 1

Why Go Dry

Whether you're a Dry Jan'er or rocking a Sober October, embarking on a Dryathalon means different things to different people—because factors like personal goals, lifestyles, and where you live and work all contribute to the experience. Even friends, family, and coworkers (not to mention pets) impact this commitment.

The reasons to go dry are endless, but since limitations exist (in both pages and time—and attention spans, to be fully transparent), this chapter will explore the most common motives to give up alcohol for one month—in this case, the month lots of people choose to begin their dry journeys: January. Rationales include:

- **to improve physical and mental health** (drop pounds and bad attitudes)
- **to free up spare time** (tackle that stack of books you've been meaning to read)
- **to take on a new challenge** (admit it: Life can be redundant, it's time to shake things up . . . without a cocktail shaker)
- **to save money** (cha-ching!).

SIDE NOTE: In a 2018 survey, nearly one in five Americans vowed to participate in Dry January— that translates to more than 65 million people!

While going dry, you may notice your social circle changing (which isn't a bad thing, necessarily), and you'll begin to recognize how alcohol affects your day-to-day life. A month without drinking will demonstrate how getting buzzed or drunk (and hungover) impacts every part of your world (and all the people around you). In addition, excessive alcohol use is the third-leading cause of preventable death in the United States, according to the National Institute on Alcohol Abuse and Alcoholism—so, beyond everyday life improvements, there's that.

REASON 1: It's a New Year's Resolution

3 . . . 2 . . . 1! When the ball drops, it's all Champagne toasts and kisses and good wishes for a happy and healthy upcoming 365 days. But the next morning is when the work kicks off. Regardless of what your goals are for the year ahead, January 1 marks a new beginning, a fresh start, a clean slate, and the day everyone attempts to lean into their wish lists of improvements. Instead of pledging general intentions to lose weight, spend less money, or be "healthier" (like everyone has promised before—admit it), reap all of these benefits and more when you pledge to forgo wine, beer, and spirits for thirty-one days straight.

REASON 2: New Year, New You

Dry January isn't like overhauling your wardrobe, dyeing your hair (or chopping it off), or taking on a different personality. (Note: If you want shorter bangs, please do not cut them yourself over the bathroom sink. This never ends well.) Dry January is a gradual change over a relatively short period. You have time to process each adjustment and learn from your individual, personal undertaking. It's about experiencing a different version of yourself—with the absence of alcohol. If you want blue hair, too, go for it. (My favorite shade is cobalt.) You don't have to choose between trendy jeans, highlights, and being booze-free. You can buy all new clothes, shave your head, *and* be sober for a month, if you'd like.

REASON 3: **Dig into Work**

After a (hopefully) relaxing holiday season in addition to that extended breather between Christmas and New Year's (if you were lucky enough to have a lull without deadlines, bosses, and coworkers—never mind interoffice drama and those redundant emails), the first weeks back can be best spent with a head-down attitude. Without the distraction of seasonal, year-end parties and going out with friends, it's time to get sh*t done! Imagine a world in which hangovers or drowsiness from staying out late on weeknights won't stop you! Kiss those unproductive mornings—and that double-order-of-espresso ritual (to hide your yawns)—good-bye! Get ready to be more alert and have a clearer head. A dry month won't just feel good, it will help you execute your work to-do list in an orderly, rapid-fire, efficient fashion as well.

REASON 4: **Save Money**

The holidays may have left your wallet a little lighter . . . and not in a good way. Buying thoughtful gifts for loved ones and obligatory presents for coworkers (and much-needed and deserved rewards for yourself) can add up. Fortunately, participating in Dry January doesn't cost much, if anything at all. Instead of buying $15 cocktails, $10 craft beers, or $10 to $15 glasses of wine, save all of that hard-earned cash and use it on other experiences, adventures, or items.

What does savings mean to you? Car payments (or a new car)? Six months of groceries? A vacation? A pet? Years of rent? By spending fewer dollars on imbibing, you can save up for that shiny new ride, more dinners at fancy restaurants, that dream trip you've been wanting to take, the doggie in the window (yes, the one with the waggly tail), or redecorating your home (or even moving to a nicer place).

it's time to get sh*t done!

If delicious dining options, seeing the world, and new home furnishings don't motivate you, then paying off credit card debt might convince you to cancel your plans to get wasted this weekend. No debt? Lucky you! Consider investing your saved moolah on something more meaningful. Invest in a company or stock that excites you, and watch it grow!

REASON 5: Surprise! Unexpected Benefits

Maybe you need a goal with concrete results. Or maybe you're the kind of person who prefers surprises. In either case, this thirty-one-day dry challenge is for you! Along with your plan not to spend money on alcohol and feel infinitely richer on February 1 (okay, maybe not, like, *soooo* wealthy, but), you also may notice—surprise!—that your pants aren't as snug. Perhaps, after saying sayonara to sangria, you discover that you're falling asleep earlier or sleeping through the night. In addition, what people often don't fully consider is the impact alcohol has on their social calendars. Leaving behind people you only vibe with while drunk can be unexpectedly liberating. More benefits (that you would have never thought possible) include clearer, healthier-looking skin. Even if you aren't vanity obsessed, there's no harm in getting rid of pimples and other pesky imperfections simply by abstaining from alcohol.

REASON 6: Challenge Yourself

Be honest: When was the last time you set a goal and followed through? Your objective might have been set last week, last month, or last year, but try to recall: Was it an open-ended goal or did you set limitations, like an end date or finish line? Having a deadline to accomplish your feat might be the best path to success (hello, February 1)—and a plan for getting to success doesn't hurt! While most physical fitness goals require time, equipment, money, and training, the act of not drinking calls on none of those things.

This challenge simply entails that you refrain from ordering a beverage, pouring a drink, or (at the very least) consuming one.

This challenge isn't strictly physical or mental—it's a little of both, with a tiny bit of societal pressure mixed in. But, whatever you think your weakness is (perhaps it's the temptation to celebrate a win at work with a bottle of wine or the habit of catching up with the crew while watching the game at a sports bar), the truth is, you *can* resist. It may be challenging, but you are capable of rising to the occasion and growing from it in the end.

REASON 7: **Get with the Trend!**

European fashion is always on the cutting edge: It's new, it's provocative, it's flashy, and, more often than not, it's inspiring (whether it's motivating you to buy that stylish blazer or that funky pair of socks). We can thank the UK for popularizing hot, trailblazing ideas in categories beyond clothing, like music (The Beatles, The Who, The Rolling Stones, and the Spice Girls), tasty beverages with their own time stamp (tea time), and guess what else? Dry January. If the history of cool, trendy Brits is any indication, they're ahead of the curve when it comes down to what's hot. It's no surprise that their Dry January tradition has spread to the Americas and other parts of the world, too.

REASON 8: **Take Inventory of Your Year**

The days of late December often inspire us to think back on the last twelve months—what have we accomplished? Who are we spending our time with? Are our finances in order? What do we want to accomplish in the coming year? And that's where our resolutions start to take shape. Some people schedule brainstorms and huddles. As you're thinking through your checklist, it's likely you'll have a drink in hand at some point between holiday parties and get-togethers.

When January 1 rolls around and Dryuary participants (like you) pledge to give up booze, an often overlooked reason to do so is for the sake of analyzing what role alcohol plays in your life. Some things to consider are who you're drinking with, how these plans originate (and how often), and the feelings you feel before and after a cocktail (or beer, or wine, if you prefer). Is alcohol a social buffer? A means to make or withstand big and small relationships? People drink for different reasons: to have fun and celebrate, to bond and to be social with others, to relax and decompress after hard days, and even to just get off the couch and out of the house.

So, after not drinking for one month—or maybe even halfway through or after one week or just one day into the month—you'll start to recognize your triggers, such as the abundant opportunities that facilitate drinking for emotional, spiritual, social, and societal reasons (including a bad day, a holiday, a birthday party, and a happy hour with coworkers). As always: no judgment. Whatever the reason for getting that drink may be, note what drinking does for you and how it functions in your life.

REASON 9: Improve Health

Joining a gym on January 1 is so cliché. Just kidding. It's awesome! And if you have a set goal, like running a 5K or riding the front row in spin class, that's amazing, too. (We'll be cheering you on from the sidelines and row two, respectively.) Incorporating healthier foods and meals into your diet is a great start to a new year as well.

Both dieting and exercising require budgeting, a time commitment, and thoughtful planning. But it's all worth it. In the end, you'll look better on the outside and feel better overall—which are also the perks of a booze-free month.

Cutting out alcohol does wonders you can't even see! Beyond possible weight loss and better sleep, the rest of your body, from your brain to your skin, benefits.

However, a Dryathalon doesn't require barbells or yoga pants (although, we think the combination of mocktails and muscles make a great team), and you don't have to count macros or spend money on fancy products that promise promoting a better physical you. Hell, it doesn't even entail leafy greens if you don't want it to. The only thing that is 100 percent necessary is taking a pass on wine, beer, and spirits.

By ditching drinks for a month (or even a night out), you're automatically cutting carbs, empty calories, sugar, and salt. If any of these elements are on your "do not consume" or "cannot eat" lists for the year ahead, consider them checked off.

REASON 10: Free Up Spare Time

The excuse "I'm too busy" isn't a new one. When people can't commit, follow through, or complete a personal task or goal they've been wanting to accomplish, they blame the responsibilities of work, family, or friends, and even themselves—too tired, bank account balances too low, a spare hour isn't feasible. Making plans with old and new friends can get pushed off for weeks—even months. But when you give up drinking, you're also leaving behind late nights, hangovers, sleeping in, and feeling lethargic the next day.

When you choose to go dry, you can still go out to bars and stay out until the wee hours of the morning (if you want to), but it's likely you'll pass on some of those opportunities and gain open evenings to do whatever it is you want to do. Instead of filling this time with shots of vodka and dancing or ordering frozen drinks that *must* be uploaded to social media before consumption, you might find yourself picking up the dusty guitar in your apartment during a quiet night at home. Maybe you'll catch up on episodes of your favorite streaming series. Instead of long dinners with bottles and bottles of wine, you'll have time to teach yourself how to make a four-course meal instead. (Watch out, Martha Stewart!)

REASON 11: Change Up Your Social Circle

Sure, friends stem from different parts of life: childhood, college, graduate school, adulthood, work, that random kickball squad you joined at twenty-two, a spring-break trip, your ex's family. . . . You get the point.

Every day and every week, you may tend to socialize with the same individuals. Most people work Monday through Friday, and lead their lives with a similar routine each day. Even the weekends may follow a pattern. In general, it's no surprise that coming in contact with the same faces on a daily and weekly basis is standard—unless there's a life event like a wedding or birthday (which are both occasions to drink, but stay focused!).

So it's likely you're imbibing with the same people, day after day, week after week, and month after month.

Without an Old Fashioned in hand or splitting a bottle of wine, is it possible to maintain these relationships?

If the answer is yes: Plan an activity that doesn't have to do with booze, like going to a yoga class together. (See page 90 for additional ideas, like traveling, eating at a new restaurant, or working out!)

If the answer is no: Without plans (and friends) that revolve around cocktails and happy hours, this is a great opportunity to reconnect with people from your past or present who don't drink at all, peers who want to do stuff that doesn't mandate drinking, or other fellow Dry January participants who are looking for cool things to occupy their leisure time.

Going to new places on any given day or night can open you up to a new crowd of potential friends with interests similar to yours—which is especially important if your comfort zone is hitting the same bars, lounges, restaurants, or neighborhoods every week. When you're not under the influence of alcohol and meeting new people, you can immediately tell if you enjoy their company (and vice versa!). Without drinks, there isn't a B.S. booze-filter encouraging fake friendships or acting as social lubrication to ease uninteresting conversations.

Now that you have multiple, motivating reasons answering why you should commit to Dry January (or any other alcohol-free month), it's time to explore what benefits you'll reap when you remove booze from your lifestyle for thirty-one days.

Gauge Your Level of Intention, Rather than Level of Intoxication

Why go dry in January, or any other month? Sometimes it can be summed up in one word. Sometimes, seven sentences aren't enough. After all, every person has his or her own reasons! This survey will measure what motivates you the most. On a scale from 1 (don't care) to 5 (must have), rate your rationales.

NEW YEAR'S RESOLUTION TIME!
I want a challenge with start and end dates.

| 1 | 2 | 3 | 4 | 5 |

NEW YEAR, NEW YOU.
I'm looking for a gradual, day-to-day change.

| 1 | 2 | 3 | 4 | 5 |

I'm digging into work and GETTING SH*T DONE.

| 1 | 2 | 3 | 4 | 5 |

I want to save MONEY.

| 1 | 2 | 3 | 4 | 5 |

MORE AESTHETICALLY PLEASING SKIN PLEASE(!),
without the makeup counter markup.

| 1 | 2 | 3 | 4 | 5 |

IMPROVED SLEEP, without counting sheep.

| 1 | 2 | 3 | 4 | 5 |

TA-TA, tough tummy!

1   2   3   4   5

I'M CHALLENGING MYSELF
(like I did that one time in seventh grade P.E. class).

1   2   3   4   5

BRING ON THE TRENDS!
I'm down to try a fad, especially if it originated in Europe.

1   2   3   4   5

I'M TAKING INVENTORY of the relationships in my life.

1   2   3   4   5

IMPROVING MY HEALTH IS A PRIORITY
(I even bought new gym shorts).

1   2   3   4   5

CAN'T WAIT TO FREE UP SPARE TIME (for uh, other stuff).

1   2   3   4   5

A CHANGE in my social circle could be cool.

1   2   3   4   5

Participating in activities MAKES ME FEEL ALIVE!

1   2   3   4   5

CHAPTER 2

What You'll Gain When You Lose the Booze

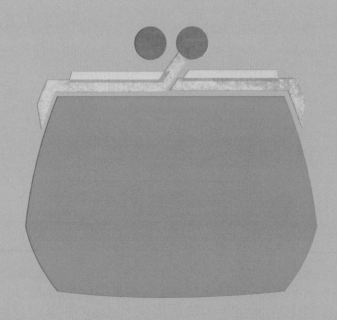

There are tons of crystal-clear reasons to jump on the Dry January (or Sober October or No-Drink November) bandwagon, but you'll discover other, not-so-obvious benefits of taking a month off from alcohol as well. You might go into this experience just expecting to drink fewer martinis, but your month-long challenge will include some surprise perks.

Case in point: Eliminating alcohol from your everyday (or weekly) routine for thirty-one days will also influence how you spend money, consume beverages and food, and occupy your time.

It might be hard to imagine exactly how your lifestyle will be different when alcohol is out of the picture, but once the bills, calories, and hours are added up, you'll never look at a drink the same way again. Numbers—just like unforgiving hangovers—don't lie!

Fewer Parties, More Pennies

From hostess gifts to ordering drinks at sports games, from buying shots during birthday celebrations to unwinding at home, purchasing cocktails during just-for-fun outings, and everything in between: The final tally spent on mixed drinks, shots, beers, and vino might surprise you. Perhaps you have a specific budget for getting buzzed (when Dry January is not in session), and you've already calculated how much you're comfortable spending at the liquor store each week or month. If that works for you, great! If you're looking to pay off credit card debt or struggling to submit a rent check each month, read on.

According to Department of Labor statistics, Americans spend, on average, about 1 percent of their annual paychecks on booze! Think about what your yearly salary is—now divide that by one hundred. What would you do with that extra cash in your piggy bank? Would you eliminate credit card debt or student loans? Maybe you'd treat yourself to that Mediterranean cruise that you've always wanted to take, or revamp your wardrobe, or invest in the stock market, or buy a loved one something he or she has always desired. Whatever your objectives are—go for it! In fact, going after your dreams makes a dry month easier to achieve.

"When embarking on a challenge like Dry January, it's best to connect it to a very specific goal you really care about," says Shannon McLay, CEO and founder of The Financial Gym, which takes a fitness-inspired approach to personal finance by pairing clients with financial trainers. "Define what achieving that goal really means to you."

McLay gives the example of, say, wanting to go on a seven-day trip to Iceland with your best friend. First, you take a peek at the price of flights and accommodations, estimate how much you'll spend on food and entertainment per day, and add that all up. Once you have a magic number, you can compare the trip's price tag to the total amount of money you'd save every day (by simply not imbibing)!

"Breaking it down makes it much easier to say 'no' to the day-to-day stuff because you're saying 'yes' to Iceland next year," says McLay.

THE RIPPLE EFFECTS OF RIPPING SHOTS

While you're working through the calculations (multiplying your weekly whiskey sour consumption by fifty-two weeks in a year), try adding up other less-obvious charges on your credit card that stem from drinking (even if you're really lucky, and the restaurant owner where you often imbibe is your BFF—Best Friend Forever, or Booze For Free homie). Drinks at the bar might be on the house (or less expensive than any other neighborhood business), but there are hidden costs to drinking that go beyond sipping vodka sodas or Sancerres.

Say your drink of choice at your favorite local bar costs $10 (which is relatively low for most cocktails). If you have two or three each night and go out three times a week, you're spending between $60 and $90 every seven days! Altogether, that equals $3,120 to $4,680 each year. That doesn't even include the tip . . . or safely finding your way home!

$3,120 to $4,680 each year on alcoholic beverages

Getting to and from imbibing spots will also have you reaching for your wallet. Driving a car or motorcycle (and even pedaling a bicycle, steering a boat, or a scooter) isn't an option when drinking is involved. A friend or loved one dropping you off and picking you up free of charge is a very sweet gesture (thanks, Mom!), but probably not regularly sustainable—especially if your ride wants to sleep before last call at 2 a.m. (Yes, some people—including Mom—prefer their beauty rest uninterrupted.)

Cabs, car services, and most methods of public transportation (whether bus, subway, train, or trolley) come with a price tag. In New York City, a one-way subway or bus ride costs $2.75, so even before you order a drink (or walk into a bar, for that matter), you're already spending $5.50 a night commuting to and from your destination. If you go out three times a week, your transportation expense (concerning alcohol-related activities) is $16.50. Multiplied by fifty-two weeks in a year? That's $858! And, obviously, if you call a car or hail a cab, it's much, much more.

Also, don't forget: Even if you're someone who drives to the bar (and leaves the car there, or has a designated driver), gas costs money, too. Even if your friends (or parents) are kind enough to chaperone you to and from places in their vehicles: returning the favor (or paying for gas) is the nice thing to do. (Alternatively, when it's Dry January—or Sober October or Dry July—you can hold the title of designated driver and cash in on favors from friends and family!)

Drinking at home involves discrete costs as well. Your wine or beer may require (or at least benefit from) fancy glassware or steins for the best-tasting pours. Furthermore, for spirit drinkers, unless your desired liquids are consumed neat or on ice, they're going to need a mixer (like cola, seltzer, or juice). And, if you're feeling creative and want to develop hands-on cocktail recipes of your own (or reenact classics), this DIY activity could require specific ingredients like garnishes and syrups and special tools, like shakers and strainers. The tab for staying in to drink can depend heavily on the quality of your beer, wine, and spirits, in addition to what each cocktail entails. Another big factor is the number of people you're serving—all of whom have to hitch a ride to your place, which will add to both your and their overall costs for the night. Even if you're not the one commuting to your friend's abode, *someone* (like your beer-pint partner in crime or your group of drinking buddies) is paying a little more! Itemize these elements, in your physical or online cart, and see them all add up!

Hangover remedies impose another debit from your bank account. The range of supplements and quick fixes (used before and after imbibing)—like tablets, liquids, and IV drips—aren't free.

Even healthy foods and drinks that you might not buy otherwise—like coconut water—can pack a hefty price tag when you add them up every week. And, let's not forget late-night munchies that can have you shelling out cash for pizza, cheese fries, tacos, and other snacks at eateries (or bodegas) that are open for business after bars, clubs, and lounges close their doors. Those dollar slices will dissolve hard-earned cash over time.

RED WINE VS. EARLY RETIREMENT

It all adds up: $3,120 to $4,680 each year on beverages and $858-plus a year on public transportation (per 2019 New York City fares) to get to and from your drinking location. Now see what happens when you multiply that over a decade. (This number will be much more if you use cabs or private cars—and the evening's tab may multiply if yummy food is involved at dinner, or post-partying. It's also important to note that this total doesn't count for the inflation of booze prices over a decade!) The cost of imbibing two to three nights a week for ten years costs between $39,780 and $55,380.

In all seriousness: Did you just gasp, text your best friend the news, and recalculate all of this? Take a deep breath. Let it out. You're probably thinking: How it could be possible that one person (you) could spend tens of thousands of dollars to get tipsy? Yes, it's true. Okay, once you've maintained a regular heartbeat—refocus, because there's more. That grand total only represents glass clinking for ten years of Prosecco and the like (not even an entire lifetime)!

Imbibing two to three nights a week for ten years costs between

$39,780

and

$55,380

As you're wrapping your head around how to spend your newfound cash (shoes, sports tickets, a vacation), consider an early retirement. Really! While saving money is often associated with fewer online shopping bills (inevitably helping your bank accounts retain a larger balance), some Americans are achieving financial independence by age fifty! Fifty!!! That means they tell their bosses "buh-bye"—nicely, of course. Want to quit your job at a younger age? A sober month can get you closer to that reality. You don't necessarily have to give up your fancy gym membership to live below your means. Instead, skipping out on a month of drinks and drunk food can help you achieve this goal.

Pour One Out for Work

While participating in a dry month can be a game changer for your personal finances, it might benefit the country's economy as well. According to a Centers for Disease Control study, drinking cost the US economy nearly $250 billion dollars in 2010. That price tag accounts for 365 days of criminal justice fees for alcohol-related crimes, as well as medical bills and lost productivity—all stemming from boozing!

Okay, so, initially this might not have a direct impact on you, right? If you take a day off here and there to nurse a hangover, perhaps you feel like it's all good. Unfortunately not. Research showed that 40 percent of the quarter-trillion-dollar bill was paid for by you, the American taxpayer. Ouch. Regardless of where you stand on politics, there's no doubt that your money (year after year) could be better spent by the government.

Weighing the Effects of Drinking

Here's a no-brainer: The new year often inspires new resolutions, some of which are more popular than others (and for some resolutions, people go all-in, commiting to transform major aspects of their lives). If January magazine covers (boasting "new year, new you" fixes), websites, and even social media are any indication, year after year, many, many people vow to "eat healthier" and lose weight. Can you still enjoy your weekly wine night and lose five pounds? Maybe. But you might achieve faster results without drinking the vino.

Common sense might tell you that in order to drop pounds one must cut calories (yes, that's true), but figuring out how to eliminate them (and how many to do away with) is a bit more strategic. Some people prefer to consume less food—and fewer drinks—or to exercise and burn energy, or do it all!

Unsurprisingly, an easy way to forgo extra calories is—you guessed it—to eliminate alcohol from your diet. Choosing not to drink for a month automatically cuts calories—without you having to think about what the lowest-calorie cocktail on the menu is. If you're curious (during the other eleven months of the year):

- **An average five-ounce glass of red wine** is about 125 calories.
- **A can of beer** totals roughly 154 calories.
- **A one-ounce shot of vodka** is 65 calories (without mixers like juice, soda, syrups, or tonic, which all can add calories to your cup).
- **A single eight-ounce margarita** can contain 455 calories— all by itself.

Using the same elements that you used before to tally the cost per week: If you're consuming two to three drinks a night, three times each week, your calorie count for alcohol alone is 390 to 1,386 calories between any given Sunday to Saturday—and a range of 20,280 to 72,072 extra calories annually.

SIDE NOTE: On the low end, 20,280 additional drink calories equals a pint of low-calorie protein ice cream per week. On the high end, 72,072 calories is the sum of energy packed into a pint of full-fat ice cream per week!

And, if you've opted for that delicious marg . . . you've added 2,730 to 4,095 calories to your diet in one week! For you mathematicians, that's 141,960 to 212,940 calories each year.

MUNCHIE MAKEOVER

Just wondering: After consuming a couple drinks, have you ever craved a healthy, well-balanced kale salad with a rainbow of vegetables and fruits, lean protein, the perfect amount of macros? . . . No? It isn't your alcohol-inspired after-meal? Don't worry—no judgment . . . really! You're certainly not alone, as you probably could already tell by the late-night lines you've waited on with friends and other customers also craving chicken nuggets, greasy pizza, and crispy fries. There are a lot of people who drink and then make less-than-perfect (in short: regrettable, drunken) decisions when it comes to meal choices and consuming them during late(r) hours. But not during Dry January, or any other dry time frame!

- **Ten juicy chicken nuggets =** 470 calories.
- **One fresh-out-of-the-oven slice of pizza =** 285 calories.
- **An order of perfectly crispy medium-size fries =** 385 calories.

If you order just one of these items two or three nights a week after drinking, your calorie consumption increases with every bite, adding 570 to 1,410 calories to your intake every week. In one year, that's 29,640 to 73,320 calories—on top of the calories you're drinking!

By simply deducting these late-night foods, you could lose twenty pounds in a year. You may be thinking, "I don't ever eat fast food when I drink." If that's true, and this advice doesn't apply directly to you: bravo! Keep reading for some interesting factoids to keep yourself from falling into the late-night munchies trap (and help your friends stay out of it, too)!

To put all of these eating and drinking calculations into action: Consider that losing one pound of fat involves burning 3,500 calories! In order to drop a pound per week, you must subtract about five hundred calories a day, each day. Passing up just one spicy, salted (or no salt), flavored (or original) margarita means you've almost reached the daily elimination goal, and that one small change could get the number on your scale down ASAP. Even if weight loss isn't part of your list of New Year's resolutions, it can organically happen for you once alcohol (and junk foods that follow) are no longer part of your weekly regimen.

> PRO TIP: IF BURNING CALORIES IS TOP OF MIND, USING UNOPENED BEER, WINE, OR LIQUOR BOTTLES AS DUMBBELLS IS TOTALLY KOSHER BY DRY JANUARY STANDARDS—AS LONG AS YOU DON'T OPEN THEM.

Cut Back on Wasted Time—Literally

Generally, whatever your drinking endgame motivation is—whether it's to party hard or take the edge off a stressful week—imbibing is rarely an activity that takes five minutes or less. Drinking can occupy considerable amounts of time (translation: hours upon hours!) throughout your days and/or nights (and weeks!). (Note: Chugging and shotgunning beers, slinging straight shots of alcohol, or even guzzling a bottle of wine if you want to—without a glass, because efficiency and sustainability, right?—will have you buzzed and/or drunk in no time . . . depending on your weight, height, and tolerance, of course. Although no one is holding a stopwatch, it's fair to say these bold acts of boozing can take just mere seconds or minutes to accomplish.)

Quickly meeting a friend for a glass of wine (or opting to venture out on your own for a solo serving) at a neighborhood bar or restaurant can seem like a social activity that isn't a time suck. However, when one glass turns into two, three, or more, soon you'll find that it's past your bedtime (whoops!).

Even when you limit yourself to one drink, the speediness of service behind the bar, the time of day, and other patrons (like your plus-one and how much he/she wants to drink), can affect your field trip's duration.

EVERYTHING LEADING UP TO LAST CALL

For the purpose of this exercise, consider any drinking-related expedition—from one-on-one gatherings to day drinking get-togethers to boozy brunches to full-on wild "live like there's no tomorrow" escapades—taking between one and four hours. If you go out to drink two to three times each week, that's two to twelve hours on a weekly basis spent with a cup or glass in hand. (This math doesn't include the time spent getting to and from your first and final destinations, or any barhopping or pit stops in between. It also doesn't add up the hours utilized to get ready: jumping in the shower, putting on makeup, doing your hair, changing clothes, or all of the above.)

Over a year, cracking open kegs and babysitting beers could rob you of 208 to 1,872 hours.

That's a lot of time that could be spent being productive, tackling pesky chores like organizing your home, getting ahead at work, prepping meals, or planning your early retirement. You can also commit all of these hours (that would otherwise be wasted) to doing other things you enjoy, like sleeping, reading books, watching movies, exercising, and cooking! And guess what? You can kick off catching up on all your obligatory to-dos—and fun activities—during your month of sobriety.

PERCEPTION, PINT BY PINT

If being more productive (and managing your time more efficiently) is a top resolution for the new year, cutting out alcohol will serve you well. "One of the key factors with time management is, of course, taking stock of that time we have and spending it wisely," says Tonya Dalton, founder of inkWELL Press Productivity Co. "In my opinion, this means spending that time on our important tasks. But, if that time feels distorted, it's hard to keep up. It's a bit like trying to navigate your way through a hall of mirrors." Dalton isn't referring to "the spins," one result of boozing that feels as though you're walking through a fun house. "While time is a set amount—sixty minutes equals one hour—our perception of time is much more fluid," says Dalton. "That same amount of time—one hour—can pass very slowly and leisurely while at the beach with a cocktail in our hands versus that exact same hour rushing to meet a deadline at work. Time has the ability to expand and stretch like taffy or it can easily contract and fly by in an instant."

With and without distorted time frames, not only do people lose hours to imbibing, but the aftermath of drinking (read: undesirable hangovers) can impact the following morning (and afternoon, and evening for that matter) as well—even when you've stopped boozing hours and hours prior. Depending on your specific situation, you can lose another unplanned one hour to twelve hours feeling sick, tired, and having to catch up on sleep. Simply, you may be unable to go to work, see friends (and family!), or take care of errands. Multiply those hangovers by fifty-two weeks in a year, and that's another 208 to 1,872 hours gone (quite literally) down the drain. (Dryuary = no drinks = no hangovers!)

Healthspan, a nutritional supplement, vitamin, and healthcare products retailer, polled two thousand people in the UK—where Dry January began—about how often they felt hungover. As it turns out, drinkers above eighteen years old (the legal age there to imbibe) wake up once a month feeling terrible due to the consumption of alcohol. To simplify: That totals 724 days in an average lifetime . . . *drumroll*: two whole years. (Math might not be fun for everyone, but it surely does not lie.) Instead of vomiting, sleeping the day away, or calling in sick to work, you could earn a master's degree, have two babies, and/or grow your hair a foot longer, in the same time span. (It's no surprise, then, that Dry January has grown more popular year after year in the UK and elsewhere!)

So choose wisely. The implications of drinking can vary widely! And so can the effects of giving it up.

Fill _in_ the _blank_

Before you start your dry challenge, and again when you finish it, fill in the blanks to compare the beginning and end of your endeavor. Complete this exercise honestly, or make it funny with a friend by asking them to write random words in the paragraphs below that match the parts of speech.

THE START OF MY DRY CHALLENGE

Today is _____, the beginning of my alcohol-free
MONTH, DAY OF MONTH

challenge—no booze for 28/29/30/31 days. My skin can best be
CIRCLE ONE

described as _____. I usually fall asleep around _____
ADJECTIVE   NUMBER

o'clock at night and wake up at _____ o'clock in the morning,
NUMBER

feeling _____. I do/do not wake up in the middle of the night.
ADJECTIVE   CIRCLE ONE

Overall, my tummy feels _____ after eating a meal. Right now, I
ADJECTIVE

eat and drink about _____ of calories each day. I weigh ____ pounds.
NUMBER   NUMBER

I spend about $____ each day/week on social activities involving
NUMBER   CIRCLE ONE

drinks! Last month, the best decision I made was

_____. A less-than-impressive thing I did was
PAST TENSE ACCOMPLISHMENT

probably that time I _____. At work, I feel
EMBARRASSING ACTION

_____. I feel I spend ____ hours each week drinking
ADJECTIVE   NUMBER

and on drinking-related activities. My recreational, drinking, and

nondrinking activities usually include _____, _____, and
VERB   VERB

_____, which make me feel _____, _____, and
VERB   ADJECTIVE   ADJECTIVE

_____. Overall, my attitude toward drinking is _____.
ADJECTIVE   ADJECTIVE

THE FINISH OF MY DRY CHALLENGE

Today is _____, the end of my alcohol-free
MONTH, DAY OF MONTH

challenge—no booze for 28/29/30/31 days. My skin can best be
CIRCLE ONE

described as _____. I usually fall asleep around _____
ADJECTIVE   NUMBER

o'clock at night and wake up at _____ o'clock in the morning,
NUMBER

feeling _____. I do/do not wake up in the middle of the night.
ADJECTIVE   CIRCLE ONE

Overall, my tummy feels _____ after eating a meal. Right now, I
ADJECTIVE

eat and drink about _____ of calories each day. I weigh _____ pounds.
NUMBER   NUMBER

I spend about $_____ each day/week on social activities
NUMBER   CIRCLE ONE

involving drinks! Last month, the best decision I made was

_____. A less-than-impressive thing I did was
VERB/NOUN/ADVERB

probably that time I _____. At work, I feel
VERB/NOUN

_____. I feel I spend _____ hours each week drinking
ADJECTIVE   NUMBER

and on drinking-related activities. My recreational, drinking, and

non-drinking activities usually include _____, _____, and
VERB   VERB

_____, which make me feel _____, _____, and
VERB   ADJECTIVE   ADJECTIVE

_____. Overall, my attitude toward drinking is _____.
ADJECTIVE   ADJECTIVE

CHAPTER 3

Side Effects May Vary

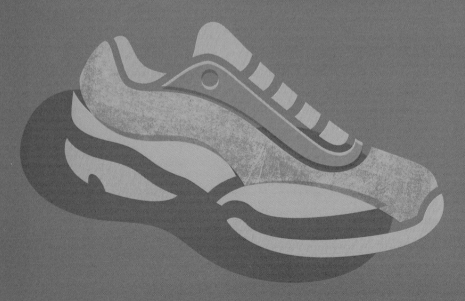

Now it's time to take a deeper look at the effects of not drinking for one month. The commitment to give up booze can inspire exercising, eating more healthfully, and engaging in other activities that ultimately make you happier. It's not just a feeling: There's scientific evidence that giving up alcohol for just one month can improve your health.

Among the pros: eating less junk food, improved digestion, healthier-looking skin, better sleep (say buh-bye, counting sheep), the ability to complete harder workouts, and clear-headedness (because who wants to be in a freaking fog all day?—no offense to San Francisco's Golden Gate Bridge). While coworkers are suffering from annoying, unwanted colds (during any time of year), you'll be cruising through your month with a healthier immune system. You'll have more energy and make smarter decisions (or at least avoid making bad decisions inspired by intoxication).

Macro Makeover

Every type of alcohol contains calories. Sugary mixes, fruit juices, and syrups—they all have calories. Every edible sweet, candied, and leafy garnish (yep, those, too) has calories. It's fair to say that most cocktail elements aren't packed with protein, nor are they high in fiber or loaded with antioxidants and vitamins—so, when you cut out booze during Dry January (or Sober October), you're cutting out tons of unneeded calories that contain little or no nutritional value (see page 41 for a calorie breakdown). Translation: If one of your New Year's resolutions is to drop a few pounds, or simply eat more healthfully, you're already one step closer to success!

"The bottom line is that if you're not feeling satisfied by the calories you're consuming, or reaping a benefit from the nutrients that food or drink contains, it's 'empty,'" says Jackie London, a registered dietitian who is the head of nutrition and wellness at WW, and former nutrition director at *Good Housekeeping* magazine. She's talking about higher-calorie cocktails—such as margaritas, daiquiris, or premade bottled piña colada mixes—and beverages made with both added sugar and cream or cream-like ingredients, like white Russians and eggnog.

But this isn't just a simple game of adding up numbers when you subtract substances—it's really about how you're consuming calories, which factors into a healthy diet and is bound to change during Dry January—or any other dry month. "When we drink calories versus eat them, we're already at a disadvantage," says London. "Chewing—and the whole eating experience—starts in your GI tract, the first organ of which is your mouth. The more you can take time to eat food you enjoy *and* get fiber from that food, the more nutritious and nourishing the entire experience becomes."

Although it's been said that drinking one glass of wine is healthy, London says there are better ways to obtain those same nutritional benefits. "With alcohol, the source matters in a way that's similar to how we think about empty calories from juice: You don't get the same benefits of drinking juice as you do from an orange, just like you don't get the same benefits of drinking wine that you would from eating a grape. Largely, that's due to fiber."

No Drinks = Better Digestion and Immunity

Are you a casual social drinker? Or a hardcore weekend warrior? Maybe you label yourself somewhere in between. Wherever you fall on the scale, alcohol can interfere with how your stomach functions. If you hate tummy aches (who doesn't?) or care about your gut health, giving up alcohol for a month can facilitate a happier and healthier belly.

"Alcohol lingers in the stomach for a while, being absorbed into both your bloodstream and small intestine," says Dr. Peyton Berookim, a double board-certified gastroenterologist in Los Angeles. "It can affect acid production, diminishing your stomach's ability to destroy harmful bacteria that enters the stomach, allowing it to enter your upper small intestine. This can also damage the mucus-producing cells

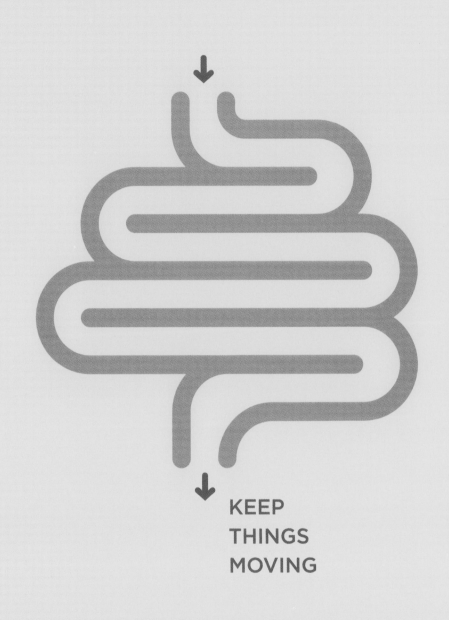

KEEP
THINGS
MOVING

that are meant to protect your stomach wall from being damaged by acid and digestive enzymes, thus inducing inflammation." Yikes! Dr. Berookim also notes that beverages with more than 15 percent alcohol by volume can delay stomach emptying, which can cause bacterial degradation of food and abdominal discomfort.

If keeping things moving doesn't motivate you, then note this: According to Dr. Berookim, booze immediately impacts the structure and integrity of the GI tract. "Alcohol alters the numbers and relative abundances of microbes in the gut microbiome. These organisms affect the maturation and function of the immune system," Dr. Berookim says. "Alcohol disrupts communication between these organisms and the intestinal immune system."

Furthermore, giving up drinking for thirty-one days straight, Dr. Berookim says, lowers blood pressure and levels of blood glucose (sugar), blood cholesterol, triglycerides, liver fats, and uric acid. Drinking elevates these elements. While blood sugar is vital for the bloodstream to carry cells and to supply energy to the body, increased glucose levels can cause diabetes, which can damage many organs in the human body. High cholesterol and triglyceride levels can lead to heart and vascular disease. High blood pressure can cause strokes and heart attacks. Fatty liver disease is linked to type 2 diabetes and obesity, and it can evolve into advanced liver disease. Lastly, gout, a type of arthritis, causes inflammation and pain, too. So, why not avoid, or at least lessen the possibility of these issues from the get-go?

If a person's levels are already sky-high, fortunately they can be lowered by participating in a sober month. "Our digestive system, including the liver, is resilient and recovers rapidly in the absence of alcohol," Dr. Berookim says.

Better Skin or Skinny Cocktails? You Decide

Vanity may not be the number-one reason you're choosing to bypass that bottle of wine during dinner; however, resisting booze will certainly help you stay looking younger. (Translation: Abstaining during Dry January can go a long way. Hey, you might actually have to bring your ID to the bar once February rolls around.)

"Alcohol is a diuretic, and by dehydrating you, it dries out everything, including your skin," says Dr. Neal Schultz, a dermatologist on Manhattan's Upper East Side and founder of BeautyRx skincare products. "By drying out your skin, you'll make it duller. You'll get more fine lines and wrinkles, which also result in shadows being cast on the skin, which makes the under eye area look darker."

Dr. Schultz notes you may not become dehydrated from drinking one glass of wine once a week, but over time it will show. Even if finding the fountain of youth isn't on your radar, there are other skin-related benefits to not imbibing. If you've ever had a pimple you *just* can't get rid of, or another annoying skin problem that can't be solved, giving up booze may be your best bet. Dr. Schultz confirms acne rosacea is triggered by alcohol consumption, so, rather than adding steps to your morning and nightly beauty or grooming regimens (with a million-plus products on the market—like face masks, cleansers, toners, moisturizers, and more), see how a month of no alcohol saves your skin!

Dr. Schultz says that alcohol increases blood flow through the skin, which gives it a red flush and ultimately causes broken capillaries. "It makes your skin look blotchy, discolored," he says. Without alcohol for a full month, an individual's skin will become smoother and less discolored. With more hydration, the skin is less dry (no flakes), and it will have fewer fine lines and reflect more light! All of these things contribute to brighter, fresher, younger looking skin.

PRO TIP: YOU CAN SAY BUH-BYE TO MAKEUP! HOWEVER, IF YOU STILL PREFER TO WEAR IT, SEE HOW MUCH BETTER AND MORE EASILY IT AGREES WITH YOUR SKIN AFTER A SOBER MONTH!

And if you think it's *just* the consumption of these liquids that's impacting your skin—think again. It's a chain reaction. "When we don't sleep well, that creates stress," says Dr. Schultz, who notes that additional hormones are produced when restful slumber goes unobtained. This, in turn, makes you break out! Also, when you aren't exhausted from a night of drinking and "too tired" to take off makeup (or simply the stress and grime from the day), there's a greater chance you'll wash your face before going to bed.

Does Booze Help Bedtime? Dream On

When was the last time you slept through the night, woke up well rested, and had a productive day? Maybe it was last night. Maybe it was last week. Maybe, luckily for you, it happens all the time! Now, think back again: When was the last time you slept through the night, woke up well rested, and had a productive day *after a day or night of drinking*? You might have a bit more trouble pinpointing a time and place! It's no surprise, then, that restful slumbers are an unexpected benefit of not imbibing.

According to researchers at the University of Missouri School of Medicine, about 20 percent of American adults rely on alcohol of some sort in order to catch Zs—or, rather, what imbibers *think* is the solution to helping them fall asleep. Ironically, that isn't the case at all. Boozing before bedtime hinders shut-eye.

Most adults need seven to nine hours of sleep, says Dr. Thanuja Hamilton, a board-certified sleep physician in Mount Laurel, New Jersey. "While alcohol itself can be sedating, the metabolism of it can cause awakenings and disrupt your sleep as your body processes it. This is the rebound effect. You may crash early on, but get lighter, broken sleep later in the night." Under the influence of alcohol, you're more likely to wake up in the middle of the night. And, because it's a diuretic, urinating more often than usual is another side effect."

Beyond waking up every so often to use the bathroom, there's yet another reason you'll be feeling tired the morning after a night out—even if you've spent a considerable amount of time under the covers: "You may initially go into a deeper sleep, but it is not a healthy deep sleep," says Dr. Hamilton. "Certain neurons/neurotransmitters are shut down, so you are less responsive, but not necessarily getting a good, deep sleep. Alcohol decreases REM sleep, so you get less of this restorative stage of sleep."

Hypothetically: Given a decision to have margaritas (which disrupt sleep) or memories (which are formed in your sleep), which would you choose? Okay. Now, apply that same question, but eliminate the hypothetical part. Dr. Hamilton says REM is the portion of slumber where dreams take place. REM is important for memory consolidation and retention, learning, and recovery. "An intoxicated person may actually spend more time sleeping, but it is the quality of sleep that is affected."

Drinking negatively impacts circadian rhythms (driven by a twenty-four-hour internal clock), which regulates sleep, in addition to other important behaviors in the brain and body. "The liver and its functioning is also part of the circadian rhythm," Dr. Hamilton says.

BREATHING OVER BOOZING

Obviously, not breathing is a big deal. You need oxygen to live! Allowing drinking to get in the way of you and oxygen . . . well, that seems like a silly choice to make. "Alcohol not only relaxes your mood but it relaxes the muscles in your airway," Dr. Hamilton says. "The collapsed contents of your throat can cut off airflow and increase snoring, or even worse, cause apneas—which is a complete lack of airflow." Breathing is vital for life (duh), so it's not surprising that restricted breaths are hazardous to your health (and existence). A less fatal, but still not ideal, side effect can include frequent and loud snoring. So, if you share a bed with your husband, wife, fiancé/ée, boyfriend/girlfriend, undefined partner, or hottie you met at the bar three hours ago, keep in mind, you may be interrupting their sleep, too, with your respiratory noises.

Choosing Happy Hormones Over Happy Hour

In the absence of boozing, and therefore late-night imbibing, you may notice that you have more energy for physical activities like exercising. Without a raging hangover and a sluggish body (and brain), you're more likely to find the motivation to get your butt into the gym (and on the treadmill or enrolled in a yoga class or whatever your preference is)!

Sometimes drinking has an adverse effect on your showing up when it really counts. Even if you keep your goals in mind, and have planned to work out in advance (like signing up for that hot new workout a day or two before), it might not happen for you—thanks to hard partying.

"In the fitness business, Sunday is the day with the highest no-show rate," says Amanda Freeman, CEO and founder of SLT, a fifty-minute studio-based workout consisting of cardio, strength training, and Pilates on a Megaformer, with locations in New York City, Boston, and Philadelphia. "Nights out and hangovers can lead to a motivation depletion. Even the greatest intentions can be sabotaged by a desire to sleep in or a splitting headache. Nights spent drinking are correlated to missed workouts."

So not only will cutting out cocktails eliminate those pesky cancelation or no-show fees (sometimes $40 a class in big cities!), actually making it to the gym (and, you know, working out) helps release endorphins. When these hormones interact with receptors in your brain, they create happy, euphoric feelings. (Yippee!)

"Lessening alcohol can be a helpful way for clients to achieve physical and emotional health because being sober helps us be more awake in our lives," says Sadie Kurzban, CEO and founder of 305 Fitness, the nonstop dance cardio workout featuring a live DJ, with locations in New York City, Boston, Los Angeles, and Washington, DC. "With exercise, we have the choice to say, 'I want to nourish my body with a workout today that gives me more energy all day! I want to do exercises where I can really stretch out some tightness because I want my body to feel more relaxed at the end of this workout.' That's what fitness is ultimately about: helping us feel healthier, happier, and more attuned to what our bodies need!"

GET YOUR
BUTT IN
THE GYM

ENROLL
IN A
YOGA
CLASS

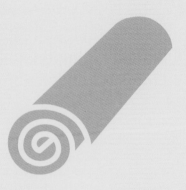

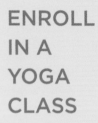

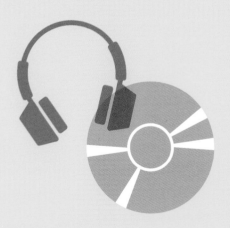

NONSTOP
DANCE
WITH A
LIVE DJ!

Employee of the Month (of Dryuary)

On the subject of being a no-show, how many times have you called in "sick" to work because of a hangover? Maybe once, maybe twice? During Dry January (or any other sober month), the answer is zero. The average working adult takes two days off every year solely to nurse his or her post-drinking ailments, according to Delphi Behavioral Group, an addiction treatment organization. (This isn't beneficial for companies that pay staff for time spent away from the office—more specifically, because staff drank too much.) Taking a day off can be good for the soul for any hardworking employee, but not when nausea, headaches, and vomiting are the cause. Upon returning to your desk the following day, having twice as much to do and playing catch-up can be stressful. Certainly, it's not the kind of welcome back you'd hope for after a day spent recovering!

SIDE NOTE: In a research study conducted by Dr. de Visser of the University of Sussex in the UK, 57 percent of Dry January 2018 participants reported better concentration.

Next work-related question: Ever go to your job hungover? If so, this definitely won't be happening in Dryuary! Save your oversized sunglasses, greasy breakfast sandwiches, and massive sports drinks for other seasons. In the same Delphi Behavioral Group poll, 75 percent of workers admitted they'd shown up to work hungover, all of them feeling the ugly wrath of being overserved. How often does this happen? About six days per person, every year. Realistically, as anyone with a pounding head can attest, it's not easy to get work done.

Every day of your dry stint, rather than popping pain relievers and chugging gallons of water at work, you'll be breezing through assignments, meetings, conference calls, and presentations (or whatever it is you specifically do to earn a living)—without painful head and tummy distractions.

With this kind of focus—hey, you might get promoted!

Memories or Merlot

Remembering your team members' and bosses' birthdays (and other important work deadlines) might help you move up the corporate ladder a bit more quickly—but listening to what they say in social situations is imperative, too.

After-work happy hours can be great for bonding with coworkers—yes, even during Dry January (order a seltzer, or a soda, and go hang)! One downside to imbibing (which you won't be experiencing) is trying to recall details of the stories and other crucial, sensitive information people tell you. Conversations with twists and turns (and multiple characters) can get a bit fuzzy after a drink or two.

The National Institute on Alcohol Abuse and Alcoholism presented research stating that people who drink a lot can experience retrospective memory loss. According to the organization, drinking heavily hinders the brain's ability to develop new memories (translation: people won't remember what happened when they were drinking). Some people call this blacking out. You won't be doing any of this during Dry January, and your friends, family, and colleagues will thank you—for your heightened listening skills.

Without booze, you'll remember more, too. And probably make better choices, as well.

Decisions Under the Influence

Following a night of drinking, have you ever woken up in the morning (or afternoon) and asked yourself, "Why did I do [insert uncharacteristic activity here]?" Been there, done that.

While intoxicated, spilling a shocking secret, spreading embarrassing gossip, streaking through a crowd, acting out, or presenting a different side of one's personality are pretty common.

Dopamine levels increase in the brain when you drink. These signal pleasure—aka those euphoric, happy feelings that ensue while sipping your favorite boozy beverage. (Yay!) Simultaneously, the prefrontal cortex decreases in activity. In short: the part of the brain responsible for rational thoughts and decision making. And, when it isn't functioning at its usual capacity or pace, thinking with clarity is unlikely.

Your inhibitions are compromised, too—leading to events that otherwise might not occur.

Following a night of drinking, have you ever woken up in the morning (or afternoon) and asked yourself,

"Why did I do _____?"

(UNCHARACTERISTIC ACTIVITY)

"We tend to regret who and how we were the next day and sometimes the damage done can destroy relationships and opportunities," says Dr. Sherrie Campbell, a licensed psychologist in Orange County, California.

Dr. Campbell notes that alcohol has a huge impact on emotions as well, which can definitely change the social atmosphere. "Whether someone changes personality by becoming a crying, sobbing hot mess, or they become angry and violent or cold and unemotional, the emotions are exaggerated," Dr. Campbell says. "When the emotions are exaggerated, they are guiding our reactions to be based in a lack of rational thought and behavioral controls."

Alcohol affects our abilities during hangovers, too.

"Hangovers cause depression, low frustration tolerance, and anxiety," Dr. Campbell says. "These emotions tend to make us needy. This neediness distorts our decision-making process."

Not consuming alcohol during January could be the first good decision toward a domino effect of other great choices throughout the year!

A Lighter Bar Tab This Year

Being more in control of your behavior and emotions during a dry month is great. What's better? These patterns and habits will likely continue beyond thirty-one days.

It's not crazy to think about extending all of the amazing benefits (inside and out) that resulted from a month of sobriety! If one month can change your skin, sleep, and so much more, consider what's possible when these benefits continue one month, six months, or nine months later (and beyond)!

But, how do you make the first move to achieving these benefits? Read on for some intel on how to do it yourself . . .

SIDE NOTE: Dr. de Visser's research found that even during months after Dry January, Dryathalon participants drank less than they did before.

More Specifically, body [snap]shots.

This is the kind of game that doesn't involve wiping off the spillage from a one-and-one-half-ounce-shot of tequila.

Draw a line to match body parts with the side effects from drinking alcohol—that will *not* take place when you eliminate alcohol from your body for thirty-one days (or any extended stretch of time, really).

1. Drinking can increase the likelihood of fatty liver disease, which is linked to type 2 diabetes and obesity. •

2. Imbibing decreases REM sleep, which is needed for memories, learning, and recovery. •

3. Alcohol, a diuretic, dehydrates the skin, making it look dull. •

4. Boozing can restrict breathing, causing sleep apnea and snoring. •

5. Alcohol affects the microbes of the gastrointestinal system and elevates levels of glucose, cholesterol, and triglycerides. •

6. High-calorie cocktails (and other alcoholic beverages) contribute to consuming "empty calories." •

- BRAIN
- SKIN
- MOUTH
- LUNGS
- LIVER
- GUT

ANSWER KEY: 1. LIVER 2. BRAIN 3. SKIN 4. LUNGS 5. GUT 6. MOUTH

CHAPTER 4

DIY
D-R-Y

Some people wake up in the morning (or afternoon) of January 1 and decide, with their New Year's Eve hangover raging and nausea at its peak, to give up drinking on the spot. Others benefit from a little prep ahead of January 1 (and also benefit from having something to get excited about as December winds down).

Will you play Dry January, Sober October, or other periods of time, on the fly—day by day—or will you map out your month and have things to look forward to? Or will your strategy involve a combination of planned outings and spontaneous get-togethers? Whatever method prevents you from taking even just one sip of alcohol, do that. The choice is yours to make. But remember: While an entire month of drink-free days and nights is the objective, it's still important to enjoy yourself (and live your life) along the way.

Your options:
1. **Be strategic about your sober month ahead of time** (translation: before the clock strikes midnight on New Year's Eve). In the December days leading up to the New Year, you can opt to toss out, give away, or hide (in unreachable places) all of your alcohol if you think having bottles around may be too tempting throughout.
2. **Develop a month-long outline** to maintain a super-fun (still dry) social calendar—or don't. Strategize how to remain strong in these social settings. Cutting ties with your drinking buddies isn't necessary, but taking the lead on planning activities that are unrelated to bars, clubs, and alcohol in general will help you feel social during what can be a cold, dreary, post-holiday blues-y month. Sometimes drafting a blueprint is the best path for success.

3. **What you share is important, too:** like who you talk to about your challenge and the platforms in which you indulge your acquaintances (or don't). Be as verbal or secretive about your challenge as you want. Whatever works for you. (Because why not do what's going to help you succeed in the long run?)

Give It Away, Store It Away, or Throw It Away— Just Get It Out of the Way

Out of sight, out of mind—right? If you're one of those people who can't stare temptation in the face (without courteously offering it a martini), make sure your living space is d-r-y. Coexisting with wine, beer, or spirits in your home can be tough. If the presence of booze isn't bothersome, then pay no mind and proceed as you normally would. You can even reward yourself with an imaginary bonus point! For the rest of the population: There are three foolproof options to ensure you don't slip up by taking the smallest swig from your home bar.

ASK A FRIEND OR FAMILY MEMBER TO STORE YOUR ALCOHOLIC BEVERAGES FOR THE MONTH

If your challenge is taking place in January, tell them you'll pick everything up on February 1—and even share a drink with them to celebrate your success! This plan gives you an opportunity to thank them for their support (once you've completed thirty-one days of no booze). If they're an exceptionally close friend, gift them your prized stash and offer to take back what they don't want. And, of course, offer to transport your neatly arranged bottles to them. After all, they're doing you a favor by lending space. Keep your items tidy, and make sure the lids, caps, and covers are secure!

PURCHASE A STORAGE UNIT FOR YOUR VINO, BREWS, AND HARD LIQUOR

Perhaps your friends and family don't have room in their pantry, garage, freezer, or cellar to take on your collection of super-fine spirits and mind-blowing Bordeaux (and truthfully, maybe you don't trust them not to drink it!). Putting your booze in a secure location means it will be out of sight and out of mouth (and mind) for a month. (And you don't have to worry about your friends or your friends' roommates sneaking sips behind your back.) The best part: At the end

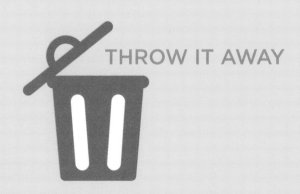

GIVE IT AWAY

STORE IT AWAY

THROW IT AWAY

of the month, you might forget what you've stored away, in which case, you'll either be pleasantly surprised when you're reunited with old favorites, or, alternatively, unexpectedly at ease upon realizing you didn't miss them much . . . or at all.

THROW IT AWAY

This might be the most controversial way to guarantee you won't be bolting for a bottle opener (and needless to say, a beer), at home after a tough or celebratory day. Pouring out expensive, hard-earned, and sought-after craft beers, exotic wines, and rare spirits (literally down the drain) might sound like a nightmare. This choice isn't for everyone—but, if you realize you still have a half-open bottle of cheap vodka from yesteryear, or two shots left of a bourbon that isn't your taste, maybe it's a good idea to clean house—if not for ridding your home of the subtle reminder that you can't drink, at least for the reclaimed real estate you'll gain in your kitchen (or other shelves in your abode).

> PRO TIP: IF DOING THIS ALL AT ONCE ON DECEMBER 31 AT 11:59 P.M. OR WITHIN THE SPAN OF A FEW DAYS (I.E., THE WEEK BETWEEN CHRISTMAS AND JANUARY 1) SEEMS OVER-WHELMING, CONSIDER BABY STEPS. EACH WEEK IN DECEMBER, TRASH, GIFT, OR STORE BOTTLES OF BOOZE. THAT WAY, IT DOESN'T SEEM LIKE YOU'RE MAKING A MAJOR LIFE CHANGE—YOU'RE SIMPLY EASING INTO IT.

While you're free to do whatever you please with your wine, beer, and spirits, it's not up to you to remove someone else's! Similarly, if your special someone or suitemates aren't participating in a dry month, now is a great time to discuss how you'll be interacting at home—more specifically, how you will not be catching up over drinks in the living room each night.

> PRO TIP: IF YOU LIVE WITH SOMEONE (A ROOMMATE, YOUR FAMILY, OR A SIGNIFICANT OTHER) WHO PRIZES THEIR BOOZE STASH (OR THEIR BOTTLES ARE MIXED IN WITH YOURS), ASK THEM FOR PERMISSION BEFORE CONFISCATING THEIR PROPERTY.

Sober Month Schedule

Planning to be drink-free from January 1 until February 1 (or any other time period) needs some ground rules. Sit down with your calendar to look at what events you already have scheduled for the month. If people will be drinking at them, decide how you're going to approach those occasions. These decisions are starting points moving you toward success.

NO PURPOSE? NO PARTY

The month of January, specifically, isn't filled with as many swanky soirees as its flashier and more sparkly neighbor, December. That last month of the year is typically jam-packed with obligatory get-togethers hosted by friends, family, colleagues, and those random groups of like-minded individuals you've accumulated over the years (from recreational kickball to book club to volunteer day and everything in between). Often there's a drinking component to catching up with these communities—whether in someone's home, a restaurant, or a bar. Who can say no to these themed outings and company parties when bonuses are just around the corner? It's true, December is a difficult month to stay dry, but by January, you'll have your (bonus) cash in hand and have caught up with all of these people. (Translation: It isn't as tough to say "see ya later" during the first month of the new year.) January has thirty-one open days of potential missteps, so it's the perfect month to cut unnecessary plans that might tempt you to order a pint . . . or two, or three. Why risk it? It might feel weird or upsetting to turn down plans and invites—but stay strong! Plus, no partying equals no awkward good-byes at bars, no polite small talk pretending you'll catch up over brunch soon, or exits without saying good night. (It's simple math . . . not drunken math!)

SAVE THE DATE (AND SPARE THE DRINKS)

If a monumental birthday, epic wedding, or a once-in-a-lifetime moment is coming up in January (in other words, it requires a formal invitation and RSVP), you definitely can (and should!) still go and have a great time without imbibing! (And really, if your best friend's sister is getting married, this is probably not even something you could realistically miss.) But, as soon as you arrive at the event, grab a glass

stay
strong!

of club soda (and some cake) to take up real estate in your hands—and belly (because, well, cake is yummy). This will not only keep you from consuming alcohol (and potentially making silly decisions under the influence), but also deflect curious questions that you don't want to answer during a celebration! (After all, this party isn't about you, it's about the guest or guests of honor!)

BE THE RINGLEADER

Friends reunite over rounds of cocktails and meet for happy hours all the time, over and over and over again. You could always politely decline and schedule a date to catch up with them during the following month, but that isn't 100 percent necessary. Take the initiative to suggest gathering somewhere off your gang's beaten path, rather than the local bar; it's a great way to breathe fresh life into a run-of-the-mill typical hangout that is expected, overdone, and no longer exciting (in truth: borrrrring. Yawn.). If your group of friends gets together every Wednesday, declare that you are in charge of picking where everyone will meet over the next few weeks. Not only will there be new scenery and opportunities to partake in different hobbies with your crew, you might also find a new regular place to spend time, even after Dryuary is over. (And P.S., even if booze is still served on-site, in places that supply more entertainment than providing drinks, you'll have an activity to focus on that will occupy your energy, thoughts, and time, allowing you to experience more than a buzz.) And—bonus points—because you're planning the itinerary, there's a guarantee you'll like what you're doing and where you're going (including the proximity to your office or home)!

If you aren't leading the pack, that's okay, too. Collaborate with the party planner or the individual who is booking that night's venue or making the reservation. (He or she might appreciate a little help!) And if things are really out of your hands, get proactive by ordering an N.A. drink before someone offers something boozy to you!

LIMIT YOUR TRIGGERS

Just like hiding booze (or donating bottles and tools to friends), you may find it helpful to eliminate booze-related reminders. Doing so may keep FOMO (fear of missing out) at bay.

After all, out of sight = out of mind.

Beyond activities and plans, consider:
- **Putting away** your bottle-opener keychains and refrigerator magnets.
- **Pausing** that monthly wine subscription delivery.
- **Monitoring** your music selection and playlists, temporarily removing songs with lyrics about boozing or popping bottles.
- **Steering clear** of sitcoms and movies that take place in bars and/or revolve around drinking culture.

STAY SPONTANEOUS

Some people are planners (hi, type A folks!), but bullet-pointing a to-do list isn't for everyone. Entertaining yourself on the fly is cool, too, because sometimes being on a strict regimen takes the fun out of your month (totally get it). Whatever works best for your personality, lifestyle, and your day-to-day life (while keeping you upbeat and happy) is how you should approach a dry month. With that said: Don't get swept away in the moment. Check in with a friend to help keep you dedicated to the goal, channel your Dry Month Mantra (take a peek at pages 206–207 for a boost of confidence), or remind yourself of that bet you made with your buddies (because you really, *really* don't want to buy them a cup of coffee every morning of February if you lose. See pages 138–139 for a friendly reminder of the wagers you've committed to). And, if you like having options but want to see how your mood is day-of, there are tons of ways to spend your time with company or alone—and certainly without cerveza—on page 106.

Spilling the (Unspiked) Tea . . . or Not

While the amount of alcohol you drink during Dryuary is definite (hint: zero, nada, zilch), the degree of how much you want to discuss your pact participation (and progress) is up to you. Like any other resolution to lose weight, work out more, save money, or commit to a new hobby, you can alert the masses, share your objectives with a few people, or keep your commitment to yourself. Dry Jan is a personal journey, and so is the choice to inform others.

Think back to a time when you took on a challenge—did you ask for support from friends and family? Or did you keep your commitment to yourself until you succeeded? (Maybe you're superstitious like that.) Whatever path of communication you choose, select the one that makes sense for your personality and will motivate you to be victorious!

NO-BOOZE BRIGADE

There's no doubting the power of strength in numbers—especially when it comes to navigating a foreign territory. Finding friends, family members, coworkers, and maybe even frenemies or forgotten acquaintances to bond over this undertaking can create common ground and an open dialogue. Relating to the same ups and downs in order to support one another can be helpful and encouraging and, most important, establish the notion that you're not alone. Your no-booze buddies can even suggest their tips and tricks to make the most of the month! And you'll probably have some ideas for them, too. More about Sober Month Support Squads later, on page 128.

CREATE, SHARE, COMMENT, LIKE!

Social media has become a major outlet for people to share and air their views, grievances, and accomplishments. Dry January, et al., are certainly not immune to this phenomenon in the age and climate of sharing experiences on digital platforms. Within these platforms, hundreds of thousands post to celebrate, humble brag, or complain about their dry progress (and why not? It's a part of their daily routines!). Whether they're uploading a photo of a mocktail or sharing a pic of their alternative activity without alcohol, some people want the world to know they're proud to be a part of this trend (and other participants, transparently, might need a "like" for an encouragement boost—no shame in that!).

The hashtags #dryjanuary and #dryjan are captioned in hundreds of thousands of posts on Instagram. And don't be fooled by less-than-positive posts that boast hashtags like #dryjanuarysucks, #dryjanuaryfail, and #dryjanuarymyarse . . . everyone's human, right?

Tens of thousands of members subscribe to the public Facebook page Dry January, by Alcohol Change UK. The wall posts focus on nonalcoholic news like tips, alcohol-free drinks, myth busters, and more. Other user-founded public and private pages and groups on Facebook promote the Dry January movement as well, allowing participants to connect with others partaking in the same thirty-one-day challenge.

Making a sober month publicly known on social channels can also help participants remain accountable, as they know the universe is watching (or at least their pool of followers . . . hi, Dad!). It can also inspire others to jump on board or supply helpful advice. On the other end of the spectrum, it can ward off enticing invites to imbibe. (With consideration and politeness: "Don't direct message me—I'll DM you!")

SECRETLY SANS BOOZE

While some participants are shouting about their no-cocktail commitments with excitement every five seconds (telling people at work, bragging to friends during recreational time, and, yes, even giving the food delivery guy the 4-1-1 about the best way to make a nonalcoholic beverage that tastes even better than the real thing), there are more discreet individuals who choose to keep quiet about their experiences. These undercover mavericks are so stealthy, you'd never know they're sipping soda water incognito during nights out on the town.

For that type of person, completing a dry month is a solo operation (and that's cool, too). Making independent choices and sticking them out can be an empowering, confidence-building experience—which only grows stronger as the days and weeks go by. You may be hesitant to announce your dry commitment to the world because of a fear of judgment (or of failing) or you just want to complete a personal challenge without random feedback. Unfortunately, these are real concerns. Outside influences (that means: stubborn friends, pestering clients, and potentially oblivious dates who don't want to drink alone) will question, tease, discourage, or tempt a Dryuaryer (or Sober Octoberer, etc.). To avoid those instances, sometimes it's best to keep your big undertaking to yourself.

There are many ways to survive (and thrive!) throughout a month without the consumption of cocktails. The point is this: If you're going to do something right, do it your way, and do it yourself (DIY)! And, on the subject of doing things yourself, it's time to start documenting your own notes during your dry journey . . .

Bookkeeping of Booze

You don't want to pour out your booze, but you don't want it in the house tempting you each and every day. To keep track of where your whiskey will have its one-month residency, here's your list of "Who Has My Booze," aka booze bookies, or friends and family who offer to babysit your Scotch during your sober month. To keep them honest, document how much is in each bottle!

If you really want to make things interesting, establish a deal: If you drink during the month, your friends get to keep your stash!

WHO HAS MY BOOZE 01

I LEFT MY BOTTLES OF

WINE   BEER   BITTERS   OTHER

WITH: _____

BRAND NAME: _____

TYPE: _____

AMOUNT: _____

BET: YES/NO [CIRCLE ONE]

WHO HAS MY BOOZE 02

I LEFT MY BOTTLES OF

WINE   BEER   BITTERS   OTHER

WITH: _____

BRAND NAME: _____

TYPE: _____

AMOUNT: _____

BET: YES/NO [CIRCLE ONE]

WHO HAS MY BOOZE

03

I LEFT MY BOTTLES OF

WINE   BEER   BITTERS   OTHER

WITH: _____

BRAND NAME: _____

TYPE: _____

AMOUNT: _____

BET: YES/NO [CIRCLE ONE]

WHO HAS MY BOOZE

04

I LEFT MY BOTTLES OF

WINE   BEER   BITTERS   OTHER

WITH: _____

BRAND NAME: _____

TYPE: _____

AMOUNT: _____

BET: YES/NO [CIRCLE ONE]

WHO HAS MY BOOZE

05

I LEFT MY BOTTLES OF

WINE   BEER   BITTERS   OTHER

WITH: _____

BRAND NAME: _____

TYPE: _____

AMOUNT: _____

BET: YES/NO [CIRCLE ONE]

Dear Dry-ary,

CHAPTER 5

"Dear Dry-ary"

There will be a world of difference between how you're feeling on January 1 (likely hungover, tired) and February 1 (more fresh-eyed, energetic). Especially if you partied hard on New Year's Eve, you'll notice the contrast without even taking notes. However, if you don't document the small details of each day, you might not recognize the reasons why you feel infinitely better.

Are you sleeping more hours each night, uninterrupted? Or exercising more because you aren't hungover? Monitoring these factors as well as your feelings, strides, and struggles can keep you motivated, accountable, and, ultimately, successful.

Documenting experiences while adopting a new plan isn't a groundbreaking concept. The same way runners track their mile times or dieters keep a food diary, try recording certain elements of each day while embarking on a sober month. Witnessing your body transform, recognizing when your mood elevates, and feeling your stress levels decrease can change your perspective about a booze-free month (for the best). It's also motivating! If eliminating just one thing (alcohol) facilitates all of these enhancements, imagine what would happen if you tuned up other parts of your lifestyle!

During your dry month, take note of information like the following:
- **What time** do you wake up each day?
- **How many hours** do you sleep each night?
- **What is your energy level** in the morning? At 2 p.m. (or whenever)? At night?
- **How is your mood** at certain times of the day?
- **How much money** are you saving by not buying drinks?

Noted: A Dry Diary, Your Way

During Dry January (or any other dry time period), it's important to track your headway (you know, and your willpower) and how you're feeling day by day. Before you know it, the month will end and you'll wonder how you got from Point A(bstain from Alcohol) to Point B(ack to Booze).

But remember, follow the method that works best for your personality, whether it's old-school scribing or new-school technology.

JOT IT DOWN IN A PHYSICAL DRY JAN JOURNAL

This old-school, classic route is best for people who want to get off their phones and computers and take a break from screen time. It's also a great excuse to go shopping, buy something new, and start another healthy habit—journaling! Note: This isn't like your top-secret middle school burn book (meaning: it's for good, not evil)! And P.S., you can share it with whomever, however you'd like (no lock and key

Before you know it, the month will end and you'll wonder how you got from Point A(bstain from Alcohol) to Point B(ack to Booze)

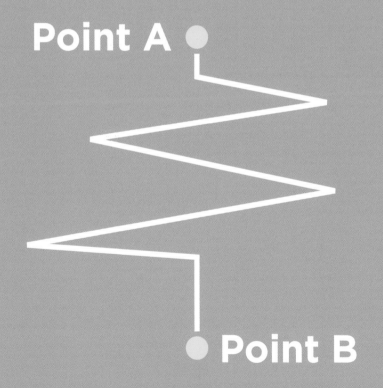

Point A

Point B

required). And don't get overwhelmed by the unlimited possibilities within the seemingly infinite number of blank pages in your new notebook, journal, or diary, either. There's no requirement to contribute thoughts every day, hour, or night—or fill every page. You can journal about not drinking as often as you please! One day, you could write five pages and another day five sentences (or five words).

Adding a bit of personality with illustrations, stickers, or doodles with colored pencils, markers, and pastels bring your entries to life (or at least make them a little bit more vibrant—if that's your style!) Get creative and channel your inner artist! The tools to document your journey lie within you (and your spiral, paperback, or hardcover log). Also, you don't have to spend a fortune on a small book with empty pages . . . feel free to scribble notes in an old notebook, a recycled notepad, or alongside your everyday journal (if you already have one)!

KEEP ACCOUNTABILITY (ALONGSIDE APPOINTMENTS)

Whether you use a datebook app in your phone or a paper agenda to keep appointments, having a space (and a steady reminder) to enter information every day can make documenting Dry January (or any other sober month) less of an annoying, obligatory task and more of a fun, easy habit. If typing or penning every day isn't for you, jot down your experiences every other day or once a week—or at random. If you're using an electronic calendar, try setting friendly, encouraging reminders to take a quick five minutes to reflect and write.

NONTIPSY TYPING

Maybe journals aren't for you (perhaps you're gung-ho about sustain-ability and you want to save paper, or just you really want to avoid paper cuts). Or, maybe your calendar is already overcrowded with tasks and to-dos. If this sounds like you, there's an easy solution: Make a special notes section in your phone to record all of your Dry Jan adventures and actions. Having a designated thirty-one-day sobriety forum in the palm of your hand(s) means you can add and edit entries whether you're relaxing on the couch, at work, out on the town, or on the go.

BLOG ABOUT NOT IMBIBING

For all you creative thinkers, designers, and writers: Try describing all your Dry January ups and downs and highs and lows on the Internet. Customizing a blog's theme, color palette, fonts, and other aesthetic elements will make this digital space feel like an extension of you. Blog about your journey in a few sentences or in lengthy paragraphs (or even haikus, if you fancy). And don't be afraid to share it with the world (or your inner circle)! Here you can update posts on the daily and make them interactive. Have commenters offer their feedback, advice, and personal experiences, as well. Of course, if you'd rather keep your entries to yourself, feel free. Regardless of who's reading (and who isn't), add personal or stock photos and other multimedia elements like links to websites, resources, and articles that are on theme with your sober month! You can post pics of your club sodas at the club or photos of activities that have replaced late nights out.

Creating your personalized online platform can be as easy as registering on Tumblr and typing away! Another option is stretching your creative limbs by using design sites with preset templates (or custom building your own), and registering a domain name to make things official. Try your first name followed by the action (i.e., [Your Name]sDryJanuary.com) or the action followed by your name (i.e., NoBoozeJanFor[Your Name].com). You can get even more creative with nicknames and other identifying elements (i.e., [Your City or State][Your Name]GoesDryInJan.com). These web addresses can be as long or as condensed as you please!

VOICE NOTES, NOT VODKA

Because intoxication won't be slurring your words, another out-of-the-box way to keep track of your shot-free stint is to record voice notes. Purchase a digital recorder, use a vintage cassette player (and tapes), or operate a phone recording app to reflect on your feelings out loud. If you have a transcription option on your phone, you can even speak into the mic and the technology will spell out the sentences for you! Organize these digital voice notes by date, topic, or mood. Play them back to yourself when you're in need of a pep talk or craving a drink, or if you want to (literally) hear how far you've come since the start of your dry journey!

Perhaps you're a professional YouTube star with millions of followers—but even if you aren't, video blogging, or vlogging, might be for you. In the same vein as text blogging, you can easily share your Dry Jan experiences with the masses or keep them more private. Whether you compile your videos online or just store them in your phone, speak openly and honestly about your sober days—allow your personality and tone to come through! You don't need a professional set, a studio, a tripod, or any other fancy-schmancy equipment to partake in homemade vlogs. Holding your camera or smartphone selfie-style, at arm's length, will do the trick. You can also ask family and friends to record you or even hop in on the action (if they aren't camera-shy and you're looking for a cohost). But for those who want to keep things simple, the best part of vlogging is that this can totally be done on your own (most cameras have a self-timer you can utilize)!

An Order of Apps and (No) Drinks, Please

And of course, there's an app—well, several—for that! You can actually take Dry January into your own hands by using a smartphone. With technology (and support) at your fingertips, reaching for your phone (instead of a bottle) can help you maintain thirty-one days of sobriety.

Dry January phone apps can track your mood, activities, money saved, and so much more! These downloadable resources are usually free of charge and help you breeze through a sober month by offering helpful tips, tricks, and reminders. Depending on your personal style, one platform may be better suited to your needs than another. You can arrange settings allowing the apps to follow up with you on a daily basis, or simply check in when it's convenient.

Developed by people who have actually experienced Dryuary (and succeeded with flying colors), the accessible tools inside these apps aren't random pointers (the content is well thought out).

It's also important to note: There are apps dedicated to giving up drinking for a period of time, and then there are platforms designed for individuals in recovery, and/or abstaining from alcohol forever. After browsing through options, figure out which works best for your needs, personality, and lifestyle, and start recording your sober month!

APPS FOR ACHIEVEMENT

Apps related to Dry January have surfaced in recent years. The official Alcohol Change UK app is called Try Dry. It helps you monitor your savings—moolah, calories, and units of alcohol—when you're no longer drinking those fine wines and cocktails or guzzling beers. Blog posts within the app are written by Dry Jan experts, too. App users can also donate the cash they save (during your streaks of days, weeks, and months of not drinking) to Alcohol Change UK. The best part of this tool is that it can be utilized year-round, beyond Dry January.

The Dry Days app also offers posts chock-full of advice (like tips for weekends) and tracks the money you save by skipping the booze (cha-ching!).

> **PRO TIP:** DOWNLOAD A FEW OF THESE APPS, AND EXPLORE EACH OF THEM BEFORE YOUR BOOZE-FREE MONTH BEGINS. THIS WAY YOU'LL HAVE TIME TO FIND THE ONE THAT BEST SUITS YOUR GOALS AND PERSONALITY. (USING ONE APP THROUGH-OUT THE MONTH WILL LIKELY SUFFICE, BUT YOU CAN USE AS MANY AS YOU WISH, IF MULTIPLE PLATFORMS SPEAK TO YOU!)

NO-DRINKING DATA SHEET

Get your geek on! As nerdy and detailed as this idea may sound, creating a spreadsheet of your sober days can highlight how booze impacts your everyday life and lifestyle. Organize topics such as hours of sleep, social activities, brain fog/alertness, and exercise (and even how many cups of coffee you need in order to get through the day). These subjects are completely customizable, so you can dictate what parts of your everyday agenda have altered. If you're completing the dry challenge alongside friends (aka your Sober Month Support Squad—more on those special people on page 128), loop them into journaling through a live spreadsheet document. As a group, you can compare and contrast your findings and update this communal chart in real time.

THE GROUP THAT TEXTS TOGETHER . . .

. . . is going to have a lot of messages pinging back and forth. Another way to incorporate friends, family, and fellow participants in your logging practices is simply by text message! While it's more informal than scribing your personal confessions into a diary, you can document and compare everything from concerns to conquests with real human beings as details develop. Assigning your text chat a creative, thoughtful name, like Daily Dry Diary, will encourage you to update your audience (whether it's one or ten people) of your progress every twenty-four hours (or so). If the title of your group message isn't enough, the text tones of other nonimbibers will also remind you to reflect on your day or week and rejoin the conversation, as well. For this method, it's best to stay away from haters who don't encourage your voyage. Instead, consult your Sober Month Support Squad for inspiration and cheering.

> **PRO TIP:** **IF YOU WORK IN AN OFFICE WITH OTHER PEOPLE AND ARE HAVING A STEADY STREAM OF TEXT MESSAGE CONVOS ALL HOURS OF THE DAY, PUT YOUR PHONE ON SILENT OR MUTE THE GROUP MESSAGES SO YOU DON'T ANNOY YOUR COWORKERS THROUGHOUT THE MONTH!**

STICKABLE NOTES

In case you forgot, here's a reminder: You've got a month of no wine, beer, or spirits! In the same way that people keep sticky notes as helpful cues taped to their mirrors, within their agenda books, or on their computer monitors, you can utilize those little sticky things to remind yourself of how many days are left in the month. As you tear the ascending days off the wall (or your desk or your refrigerator or the corner of your computer screen), write down how you feel on the back of each note. Keep these informal entries. Store them in a drawer or leave them in plain sight. At the end of Dry January (or Sober October, Dry July, or No-Drink November), you'll have a collection of tiny papers with your thoughts from each day. This is especially fitting if you don't want to wax poetic about your challenge, because these small sticky papers aren't large enough for your entire life story . . . which you'll be experiencing with fun, cool, outside-the box activities (see page 106)!

MID-MONTH CHECK-IN

Okay—so, maybe writing stuff down isn't your thing. Expressing feelings, whether via text, video, blog, what have you, isn't natural for everyone. Some people learn to love it, while others adopt the habit and do it just because. If documenting your mood, exercise, and activities, and counting your sleeping hours, are actions that irritate, annoy, or keep you from ultimately reaching your drink-free goal, then don't keep track so religiously. It's better to let something like journaling go by the wayside than sacrifice your commitment to (as long as) thirty-one days of sobriety—if January is the time frame of your challenge. Try a mid-month check-in to analyze your progress, rather than a daily, weekly, or every-couple-of-days routine. You can write down every single difference you've noticed in your body, mind, and social life, or pen a few scribbles or recite a sonnet if you're inspired.

> **PRO TIP: ON THE SUBJECT OF ODES TO DRY JANUARY: ON THE FIFTEENTH OF THE MONTH, WRITE A POEM (OR MAYBE JUST A BULLETED LIST) ABOUT ALL OF THE NONIMBIBING ADVENTURES YOU'VE ALREADY TAKEN AND PLAN TO TAKE BEFORE FEBRUARY 1!**

There's no doubt that fun, cool things to do—that don't involve getting wasted—will also play subtle and starring roles in your diary. Need inspiration on how to document your month? Turn the page for ideas.

From Sunrise to Sunset, sans Alcohol

You don't need to learn calligraphy to tally the thousands of ways a dry month changes your day-to-day life. (But if fancy, next-level cursive is your thing, go for it!) Documenting how you feel during these thirty-one days can be as minimal as a few words or as long as, um, this book. If you can't decide on a medium (journal, calendar, sticky notes, blog) to help you record the entirety of the month, get started with this chart! Fill in the blank spaces every day or once a week or once midway through the month, or whenever it fits your schedule!

INSERT MONTH HERE	WAKE-UP TIME	HOURS SLEPT	MONEY SAVED FROM NOT BUYING DRINKS	EXERCISE TYPE AND DURATION	FEELINGS/MOOD :-) - GREAT :-| - SO, SO :-(- BAD	ENERGY LEVEL 0 = FALLING ASLEEP 10 = WIDE AWAKE AND THRIVING!	DRINKS CONSUMED
1							
2							
3							
4							
5							
6							
7							
8							
9							
10							
11							

INSERT MONTH HERE	WAKE-UP TIME	HOURS SLEPT	MONEY SAVED FROM NOT BUYING DRINKS	EXERCISE TYPE AND DURATION	FEELINGS/MOOD :‑) - GREAT :‑| - SO, SO :‑(- BAD	ENERGY LEVEL 0 = FALLING ASLEEP 10 = WIDE AWAKE AND THRIVING!	DRINKS CONSUMED
12							
13							
14							
15							
16							
17							
18							
19							
20							
21							
22							
23							
24							
25							
26							
27							
28							
29							
30							
31							

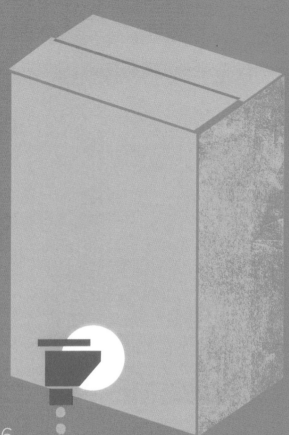

CHAPTER 6

Thinking Outside the Box(ed Wine)

In January and October, you've got 744 hours in the month to fill any way you'd like, other than with the help of, a focus on, or consumption of alcohol. Yes, a lot of that time will be spent working or snoozing (and hopefully not sleeping on the job). The remainder of your waking hours that isn't dedicated to errands, personal/familial responsibilities, and taking care of yourself, should be enjoyable, social, and relaxing!

"Going for a drink" is a standard activity for bonding with coworkers and friends. And opening a bottle of wine and enjoying solo time in front of the TV, submerged in a bubble bath, or on the couch with a book in one hand and vino in the other are common pastimes. Perhaps, like many people, you've gotten into the habit of using a glass of Pinot, a shot of whiskey, or a cold beer to unwind from the day. But all of these moments can also be achieved without a boozy touch—and just as easily, with the same relaxing benefits.

Flip the script in your head, and then in real life. Not everything (social or solo) has to involve booze—and some moments, to be honest, shouldn't! You can make the most of your nonworking, nonsleeping, no-obligation hours (whether they're slivers of time or elongated mornings, afternoons, and evenings). During any dry month, if adopting new activities makes sense for your personal lifestyle, do it! But don't forget about revisiting old pastimes of yesteryear. Whether it's a planned distraction or an easy pick-me-up, do the things you don't usually make time for and, most important, that make you happy (and keep you dry)!

Adventurous Eating without (Cooking) Wine

Approach food-related activities with as much zest as you did before you kicked off your month-long challenge. Food and drink are often paired together at fine restaurants and marketed as complementing each other; however, that doesn't always need to be the case. An alcohol-free month is the perfect opportunity to taste and enjoy your food without the influence of booze. Sometimes, people unexpectedly eat more in a tipsy state (cue: overindulging), and they miss out on subtle flavors because they're preoccupied with taking the next sip. In order to avoid the temptation of a meal with a perfectly paired wine list, you can cook at home for yourself and others, crafting new recipes or following those found in cookbooks or on the Internet. Plenty of YouTube videos provide step-by-step instruction, too.

When you're snowed in (if the temps drop low), or simply don't want to bear the cold outside, Dry January is a great time for testing out different types of dishes with a variety of ingredients from far-off destinations, or those that are compliant with all sorts of specialty diets. (Find hungry helpers to sample your stuff—they might even volunteer to pick up half of the grocery bill or assist with cleaning dirty pots and pans following your experiments.)

PRO TIP: CHEW GUM OR DRINK FRUIT JUICE WHILE YOU'RE HARD AT WORK IN THE KITCHEN—REPLACE THAT GLASS OR TWO OF WINE YOU USUALLY CONSUME WHILE CHOPPING ONIONS AND DICING TOMATOES. MOCKTAILS ARE ALSO APPROVED AS ON-HAND BEVERAGES.

Friends and family don't have to be just spectators (or taste-testers), either. Have them pitch in with their individual skill sets as sous chefs. Know someone who makes a mean meatless meatball? Ask him or her to teach you how. Or host a handful of people at your place and arrange a potluck breakfast, lunch, dinner, or brunch. Having people contribute by bringing their own dishes is an easy way to get everyone involved without too many cooks in the kitchen (and that way everyone also contributes financially to their share of the pie—literally)! And if

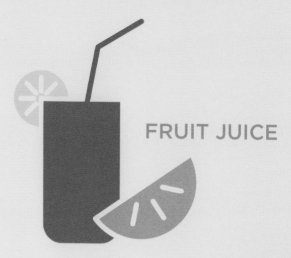

FRUIT JUICE

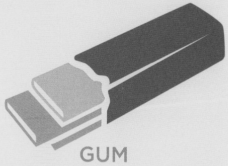

GUM

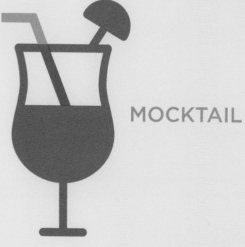

MOCKTAIL

your clique isn't super skilled when it comes to utilizing spatulas and shredders, encourage newbies to join in with basics like mixing, mashing, and measuring ingredients.

If your culinary skills aren't already on par with *Top Chef* (IRL: the microwave is your BFF), branching out of your comfort zone and using the stovetop or an oven might be exciting and challenging enough to keep you inside all month and out of bars. If your kitchen space isn't fit for cooking up a storm, look into cooking classes. In big cities, there are venues with designated spaces for teaching novices and pros how to perfect everything from bagels to Bolognese. These one-time and reccuring sessions might require you to sign up in advance, and they can be done solo or with a group.

If cooking is simply not for you (because donning an apron and measuring ingredients is really not your thing), get out of the house to nosh at a local restaurant. Old favorites or new eateries—or least places that are new to you—will do!

THE CREPE, CROISSANT, CAKE, CONES, AND COFFEE CHECKLIST
Before the dry month kicks off or when the mood strikes (when you really want a drink), make a list of neighborhood bakeries, coffee shops, ice cream parlors, and restaurants that you've been meaning to try with friends (who also might have some fantastic

recommendations). A few good places to start your research are blogs, social media, or search engines. Keeping this hit list handy will keep your hands off booze.

Exercising Your Right to Remain Dry: Trading the Bar for Barre

Point blank: Drinking can be a waste of time. One minute, it's 9 p.m. and you're ordering your first cocktail. After a few more rounds, shots, and socializing, suddenly it's 3 a.m. After a late night, a lot of drinks, and drunk food binges that don't exactly comprise green juices and carrots, it's no surprise you might feel like garbage up to twenty-four hours later. With a regimen like this, even the most fit athletes (or seasoned drinkers) are less than eager to wake up for an early morning jog, and certainly fatigued bodies are less inclined to bolt for a bootcamp class later on in the day, too.

Turbocharge the other popular, clichéd New Year's resolutions to "be healthier" and "lose weight" by substituting hours dedicated to working out for the hours you would have spent imbibing (i.e., consuming calories rather than burning them). By joining a gym, you can access weights, cardio machines, and a variety of other equipment to assist you with your goals—and, pending hours of operation, you can exercise when it's most convenient for you (or when you feel the urge to drink)! Some gyms have personal trainers and group exercise classes, too, so you can find your own rhythm, or work out with other people who share the same motivated outlook.

Beyond a traditional gym format (where you might be going at it alone), boutique fitness classes are perfect for people who enjoy exercising with others (much like a bar that's full of like-minded people). Studios for spinning and cycling, Pilates, barre, dance cardio, running, bootcamp, HIIT (high-intensity interval training), yoga, and more cater to communities of individuals looking for group instruction. The thirty- to ninety-minute sessions typically come with stimulating music, teacher guidance, and, for those who need a little inspiration to get through the month, mantras for extra support.

Gym memberships and classes (even packages) can get pricey, but adopting a workout routine doesn't have to cost a fortune—or really, anything at all. Pull up an exercise video online and you can have one-on-one sweat sessions at home. If you have enough self-control (and haven't hidden your booze or stored away muddlers and cocktail mixers with friends), remember: you can use wine and liquor bottles (and beer cans) as hand weights! Other accessories can act as markers for how far you need to bear crawl. And your shaker? Now it's a stylish water bottle. Additionally, if the weather is nice where you live (in short: not blizzarding), go running outside, walk in a nearby park, bike around the block, or even schedule a hike (if that's available to you).

Swapping Shots for a Spa Day

Before your dry month has concluded, treat yourself to rest and relaxation with spa-administered or at-home beauty and grooming treatments. (Whether you've gotten through dry day Number One, or have one more day to go, you deserve it!) Professional beauty appointments include everything from hair coloring to massages, facials, mani/pedis, and acupuncture—the key takeaway is that you're spending time and energy on an activity that you can enjoy and also isn't alcohol-based. (Don't forget to kindly pass up that glass of Prosecco at the spa if it's offered!) Of course, a hefty pampering pricetag isn't necessary for a day or a quick hour of self-care. You can visit your local drugstore and buy supplies to give your feet a scrub and a refreshing pedicure or purchase a pack of facemasks and apply moisurizing sheets on the cheap!

Getting the Gang Together

Although it's a very personal challenge, Dry January isn't typically a solo sport. True, you could lock yourself in your home to avoid the temptation of drinking, but that's unreasonable, and, quite frankly, completely unnecessary. When it's time to get together with family, friends, and acquaintances, there are a number of fun things you can do with your clique.

Bowling is a game that doesn't have to involve booze. Unlike sports that take practice, rolling a ball down an oiled lane to knock down pins is something people of most ages, sizes, and intelligence can enjoy (even if bumpers are involved). As a hands-on group activity, bowling allows players of all levels to chat in between their turns.

Like bowling, billiard halls can be almost synonymous with beer and booze. But without these inebriating elements, you'll have better focus, and your pool strokes and overall game might improve. Give it a shot (without the vodka shots) and see how your score adds up!

Bingo is a game regularly played on cruise ships with participants double-fisting sugary daiquiris and piña coladas. Another popular rendition is the drag-queen, showy version with big hair, dramatic makeup, and sky-high heels, often held in metropolitan cities during night-club hours (with night-club beverages). But if you ditch the tropical beverages on a cruise ship or the glitzy Cosmopolitans, bingo is a game everyone and anyone can play (even in daylight, and with the fam). So call up Mom and Dad, Grandma and Grandpa, and your younger cousins, too, to get the entire family involved for some age-inclusive fun. You can gamble or play for the sake of winning, but beware: It can get crazy competitive, especially when it's time to yell,

"Bingo!"

If you have stage fright, karaoke—an activity that usually involves imbibing—might require a shot of confidence, rather than liquid courage. Belting out your favorite pop song is as entertaining as it is liberating, so this is a great group excursion that can help release workweek (and other) stresses. Requesting sing-alongs and performing to tunes ranging from rap to rock and everything in between can be both a participant and spectator sport.

Competitive individuals who like to play or face-off during video and fair games can grab some tokens or coins (or cash) and head to the nearest arcade. Fast-paced rounds and levels keep hands occupied with buttons, controllers, and joysticks—essentially, no time to hold a beverage! From classic, well-known character narratives to high-speed car chases from behind the wheel as well as pinball, Skee-Ball, and more, challenge your friends and other gamers to (virtually) duke it out or team up to win prizes (like those cute stuffed animals)! Don't feel like spending an extra few dollars? Invite friends over to your home, if you have a video game console and controllers at home.

Outdoor Activities without Alcohol

Going outdoors will provide a breath of fresh air—literally.

For states that have winter and fall temps above 70 degrees, Dry January and Sober October are perfect times to spend an afternoon kayaking, surfing, or paddleboarding. Lounge by the pool for a lazy day (and a tan) or have a swim at the beach without daiquiris or piña coladas. Need-for-speed junkies can find their fix jet-skiing or waterskiing (granted, you need a boat, a driver, and the equipment for these more daring activities).

Should you find yourself faced with a January snowfall, building a snowman or making snow angels is a childhood pastime worth revisiting during your month-long commitment. Get creative by decorating faces on each of these wintry creations, and dress them up, too! When you return inside, instead of a hot toddy or spiked cocoa, treat yourself to a hot tea or hot chocolate to warm up.

In all kinds of weather, farmers' markets pop up around the country for consumers who want to buy local produce, fresh meats, and homemade baked goods. While most have brand names you can't find in chain grocery stores, many also sell a number of foods (such as hard-to-find fruits, obscure veggies, and specialty meats and milks) that aren't typically offered in commercial retailers either (and stuff you can use while cooking solo or with company at home). Walking around markets to visit these small vendors will give you a chance to stretch your legs during a short stroll and grab a yummy snack. The experience will also give you an opportunity to meet with farmers, purveyors, and families of small businesses that have been passed down from generation to generation, and you'll discover new farms in your area—some of which you might be able to visit in person. Which leads you to exploring . . .

New Destinations, (Still) No Drinks

In December, airline prices around Christmas and New Year's can get pricey—with crowded airports and impatient, overtired travelers whining over canceled connections! In January, traveling is usually a little less dramatic, and with fewer holiday-themed commitments like dinners, drinks, and parties to keep you pinned down, it's easier to skip town and not feel guilty about missing out on events.

Visiting a far-off place (whether a new country, state, or city) can open up your eyes to different foods, cultures, and ways to have fun without ordering a drink. Begin by brainstorming destinations with family, friends, and dry-month participants (or plan to go solo). Next, research things to do, places to eat, and how to get there. Lastly, plan an itinerary and book your tickets and accommodations.

PRO TIP: IF YOU KNOW YOU MIGHT CRAVE A CASUAL COCKTAIL WHILE ON VACAY, LOOK INTO PLACES THAT BAN BOOZE OR DESTINATIONS WITH CULTURES THAT DON'T CONSUME A TON OF ALCOHOL.

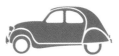

While boarding a plane for vacation sounds like a wonderful idea, jumping in the car and road-tripping can be just as exhilarating (especially if it's spontaneous). Make a playlist of songs to sing along to while driving, and pack tasty snacks for in between meals. If you'd like, recruit a copilot to take with you on your adventure. Best of all, you won't have to worry about who's going to be the designated driver. Clearly, you're not drinking on this trip!

Visiting a new place, near or far, is a lot of fun, but if you don't have the time (due to looming deadlines and other responsibilities that won't allow you to escape for too long), you can still discover an unfamiliar part of your own town—or a nearby one—and spend a day, or even a few hours, exploring.

One-Shot (Events, That Is)

Seeing an old band, a new artist, or discovering performers (and new venues) are other fun ways to spend evenings and weekends instead of barhopping. Tons of popular musical and entertainment acts tour throughout the month of January (and obviously other months, too), and their schedules are usually posted way in advance so you can plan your days accordingly. Even if you don't live in a large city or near a metropolitan area with large stadiums and arenas, look into hubs with smaller stages—even coffeehouses with local acoustic guitarists, jazz bands, comedians, and poetry readings. Without a beer in hand, you can still relax or get revved up—whatever your concert style may be.

Just like pop and rock stars, Broadway shows and other performances (dramas, comedies, musicals, and more) tour the country. There's no need to book a train or flight to New York City to check out the year's hottest stars on stage. (But, hey, if you're in Manhattan, you can see these acts in the Theater District and catch a glimpse of the bright lights in Times Square!) Bring a little bit of culture into your month, without visiting the concession stand for a drink.

SIDE NOTE: Daybreaker—a pop-up experience that involves early morning (6 a.m. to 9 a.m.) dance parties with music, dancing, and not an alcoholic beverage in sight—has spread to twenty-five cities including Boston, San Francisco, Los Angeles, Philadelphia, Amsterdam, and London since its inception in 2013. The movement was dreamed up by two friends over late-night falafels in Williamsburg, Brooklyn.

Art shows, galleries, and museums are other options for passing the time with a cultural experience. Many establishments don't allow food or drink on the exhibition floor in order to avoid any spillage and mishaps, so there's another reason to leave your thirst and flasks at home!

Pop-up festivals and expos come and go for a day, a weekend, or a week. These spectacles are often interactive and typically related to food, art, history, or heritage. Some encourage or even require a costume. (If it's a culinary event, wear your stretchy pants.) If the incredible photo ops don't convince you to attend, there's always an opportunity to eat, observe, learn, or buy something new. (But not a new boozy beverage . . . no whiskey festivals, please!)

If touchdowns and three-pointers are of interest, professional and college football and basketball seasons run through January. Some universities (like Brigham Young University in Provo, Utah) are dry campuses, meaning you can't bring or buy booze at sporting events, anyway! First downs and layups aside, these two aren't the only sports to check out during your sober days.

Instead of "skating" on slushy, dirty pub floors, watch the pros skate, shoot, and score on ice. National Hockey League games are also scheduled in January—so puckheads, rejoice! Cheer on your favorite players during this fast-paced and energizing sport. (Promise: Your clean sneakers and dress shoes will thank you later.)

Homebody Haven

Winter is the perfect season for snuggling up on the couch and binge-watching TV shows and having movie marathons. When it's frigid outside, you can be all bundled up, comfy, and warm and have endless hours to delve into character dramas, romantic comedies, scary plots, and so on. Tissues are totally acceptable during heartfelt films and series, but wine, on the other hand, is not!

Meaning to find time to finish that book you started ages ago? Pick it up again! In need of a new novel? Visit the bookstore, library, or shop online for books! You can even make reading a social event by joining a book club (in person or online) or starting one with friends, and it will keep you accountable for staying on track and completing chapters.

Drinking games have their place and time, but not during a dry month. Board games and card games are other avenues for being social, competitive, and staying out of bars! Dust off the Monopoly and Scrabble boxes for a long night ahead with company. Opt for Connect Four or checkers if your attention span is a bit shorter. Playing solo? A deck of cards and a game of solitaire will keep you occupied on your own. Even wintry, cold, dark nights can be cozy when you disconnect from electronics and engage in games that aren't on your phone, computer, or tablet.

Drinking has become a habitual part of achieving relaxation or sedation for many people looking to take the edge off from startling, unnerving, and less-than-pleasurable experiences accumulated during their days, weeks, and months. Home cocktail hours and even nightcaps (to assist in falling asleep) become the norm. Rather than making a drink disappear, try meditation. It's a practice that (for some) can be tough at first, but once you adopt a regimen that suits your needs, meditation can help you focus and achieve mental clarity and a sense of calm. Don't know how? Power up your computer or phone and search the web (or app store) for step-by-step instructional guides that will help you breathe through meditative exercises. You can totally do this at home, creating a sanctuary of peace in your living room or bedroom!

Speaking of rooms in your home: As you're figuratively redecorating your lifestyle (and replacing boozy accessories with other interests), Dry Jan is the perfect time to rearrange furniture and decor. It's also an opportune season to throw away old, unnecessary things (considering all your new, flashy holiday gifts are likely also occupying precious square footage). The bar cart that was once a centerpiece for drinking at home isn't serving the same purpose this month. While it may support your needs in February (and beyond), it's a starting point to uncovering what items can stay and go. Perhaps move this glorified storage unit to a place with less foot traffic—maybe give it to a friend (to keep or borrow), or toss it altogether. A dry month is a better time than ever to take inventory of the furnishings of your abode (and life!) that are simply taking up space.

PRO TIP: **FOR BONUS POINTS, SELL YOUR GENTLY USED ITEMS FOR EXTRA CASH OR DONATE TO NEARBY CHARITIES TO HELP THOSE IN NEED.**

Wine-and-paint nights have become popular in metropolitan cities and during private parties at designated venues. During these sessions, students can make masterpieces with a paintbrush in one hand and a glass of vino in the other. However, arts and crafts, including those involving brushstrokes, certainly do not require a boozy component or

KEEP
CALM
AND
REDECORATE

a professional studio space. Keep your creative juices flowing with a collaboration of N.A. beverages and art projects—such as painting, drawing with colored pencils or crayons, quilting, pottery, photography, and sculpting—at home! A trip to the art store will satisfy your shopping list of art supplies (and cleanup materials, so you don't ruin your favorite carpet). Especially if you're redecorating your living space, you can make your own art as you commemorate your dry month!

Giving Back (When You Give Up Booze)

When you eliminate beer, wine, and spirits from your diet, you will notice a difference in how your body and mind feel. To extend those positive vibes to others, consider giving back to the community and taking part in activities that don't allow you to drink on the job. Local soup kitchens, homeless shelters, animal shelters, and other nonprofit organizations are often looking for volunteers to help serve attendees, organize paperwork or equipment, and assist staff on-site. Drinking is typically not part of the gig (read: not allowed and not appropriate), so you don't have to worry about being offered a beverage (even as a thank you for hours of unpaid work).

Praise a Booze-Free Perspective

If you feel as if you have lapsed and are looking to return to your faith (or perhaps curious and eager to find a new direction), dry month participants can also avoid drinking by attending religious services. Different times, days, locations, and sermon focal points offer endless outlooks and opportunities to explore your thoughts and feelings about many subjects—and also open you up to social circles you might not otherwise encounter in your day-to-day life.

During this month, practicing individuals can become more involved within their communities by participating in religious study or discussion groups, assisting with fundraisers like bake sales, or volunteering for admin work (such as writing newsletters or answering phones).

The Family That Forgoes Drinking Together . . .

Before (and after) a dry month, time spent at a bar is more likely to be in the company of friends and coworkers than family. With friends: ragers, celebrations, birthdays, catch-ups, and spontaneous outings are often accompanied by drinks. With coworkers: team-bonding activities, gatherings, after-work drinks, and happy hours can cloud your weekday calendar (and weekends, too). Family time (and drinking) may not be in the mix as often, but, if it is: Know that you can see your fam without having an alcoholic beverage (though admittedly, sometimes it's easier to handle Mom's nitpicking questions if you have a glass of wine). With your parents, siblings, cousins, and other relatives (maybe nieces, nephews, and grandparents), start regrouping by organizing one night a week to bond. Dinner, casual hangouts at your home, or any other idea from this chapter will do!

Beer, wine, and spirits galore aren't a prerequisite for having an amazing night out (or in) with friends (or alone). This chapter's suggestions will keep you entertained, help you stay on track, and manifest the most fun with your social circle, new friends, and relationships from the past—minus alcohol.

A Month of Activities, without Alcohol

The thirty-one days of suggested stuff to do in this month-long calendar isn't mandatory (unless you're an alcohol-free extracurricular overachiever). Consider it a guide to not getting drunk. You can fill in nondrinking activities on your own, or take some hints from the list!

1 Hide your booze and make a bet	2 Watch a movie	3 Go bowling
8 Call a relative	**9** Paint a picture	**10** Go out to dinner

11 Start watching a TV series		

15 Remember to journal about your dry month—you're halfway there!	**16** Find a local comedy show or concert	**17** Bake cookies
22 Try meditation!	**23** Revisit an old pastime like playing guitar	**24** Go see a professional (or local team) sports game

25 Plan how you're going to celebrate at the end of your dry month!		

29 Go on a hike (or a walk). If it's too cold, stroll through a local mall	**30** Play virtual golf, or go to the arcade	**31** Organize a poker night or card game

4 Invite friends over for mocktails	**5** Go to a museum	**6** Read a book	**7** Plan a trip
12 Try a new workout class or YouTube yoga	**13** Bake a cake	**14** Go out for ice cream (or learn how to make it)	
18 Call a friend	**19** Clean out your closet	**20** Make a three-course meal	**21** Invite friends over for board games
26 Stroll through a farmers' market or take a day trip somewhere nearby	**27** Check out a local coffee shop you haven't tried yet	**28** Volunteer in the community!	

ALTERNATE IDEAS:

*Play in the snow (if you live in the North)

*Kayak or jet-ski (if you live in the South)

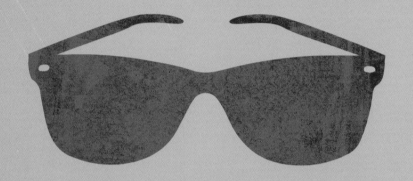

CHAPTER 7

All the Cool Kids Are (Not) Doing It

The decision to give up alcohol is a personal one and, as you can imagine, motivations differ from person to person. Friends and family might not be able to relate to your personal goals—whether those finish-line dreams are tied to health, socializing, or a simple curiosity about how alcohol affects you within a designated period. Feeling pressured, pestered, or challenged by unkind remarks (or being straight-up disrespected) isn't easy. (Stay strong!!!)

Thankfully, there are a number of ways to approach agonizingly awkward situations . . . while keeping cool, calm, and collected—and, most important, without giving in and taking a swig.

First, a Pregame Pep Talk

Have a heart-to-heart with yourself.

> PRO TIP: A MIRROR ISN'T REQUIRED TO GIVE YOURSELF A CONFIDENCE BOOST, BUT CERTAINLY CAN BE UTILIZED.

1. **Stay focused. Stay relaxed. And stay dry.** Any night out (or even at home) will be a potential opportunity to have your commitment questioned. In the face of persuasive individuals (e.g., a best friend or bartender, or a cutie at the bar), sometimes answering why you're not drinking is more difficult than actually not drinking. But you'll be prepared—you knew this was coming. Snarky remarks, side-eyes,

and judgey looks won't sway you. Handle these with grace and a smile. Tell yourself not to give in, not to give up, and not to accept that vodka soda.

2. **Allow your committed and powerful inner voice** to supply positive affirmations and lead the way. At first, people will want to know why you're doing it (which you know the answer to—see page 22 for a quick refresher). Then, they'll ask how you're doing it (no cheat sheet necessary). As the weeks fly by, their curiosity (which once seemed super judgy) now feels encouraging. Follow-ups like "How's it going?" and "How do you feel?" will start to feel like cheerleading instead of criticism (read: eye-rolls not included).

3. **Passing up opportunities to booze with buddies** is difficult the first few times you say no, but it gets easier. It gets better. It becomes a habit. Like building a muscle, your willpower will only grow stronger over time. Now, get out there and show them what you've got!

Pass on Pinot and Peer Pressure

If someone offers you a drink (at a party, dinner, or bar), politely decline—with or without explanation, depending on how you want to play it. "I'm good," is usually a nice enough response for anyone (drinking or not) to pass on a round of cocktails. You could lie and say, "I've had enough for the evening." (Lying not recommended. Tell the truth unless it's completely unbearable.) By staying honest and angelic, you are a more trustworthy and morally sound individual—not to mention that your role as a designated driver is another legitimate (and life-saving) reason not to drink as well!

What do you do if people continue to offer you a drink or tease you about not drinking? There's no reason to sink to the level of your bullies. Making a scene, becoming outraged or angry, or storming off (out of a public or private space) is not the best way to handle yourself. Hand that beer, wine, shot, or craft cocktail back to the person who purchased it. Or grant it to a friend, or set it down on the bar, table, or countertop closest to you. (And smile! You're doing great!) Bonus points: Find a cutie in the venue and gift it to them instead. (See? Dry January brings people together!)

I'm good.

I've had enough for the evening.

OR

tell the truth!

Explain Yourself . . .

The first few times you describe Dry January (or whatever month you're abstaining in) and what it means for you, the conversation may make you feel uncomfortable, because it's personal. Feeling vulnerable is totally normal. Don't be intimidated by awkward silences and an audience of furrowed brows. Relay your plans in an upbeat, excited, and positive fashion.

It's important not to point fingers and tell people why *they* should give up booze. (Just as you don't want to be talked out of your dry days, they don't want to be told not to drink.) There's a fine line between being respectful or positive versus boastful or preachy. Rest assured: You will learn to strike that balance and the conversational weirdness will subside over time. In fact, the more you resist temptation and recite your reasons (internally to yourself and externally to the people around you) in a happy tone, the more self-assured you'll become.

You certainly do not have to convince people why this is the right thing to do (or that they should partake in twenty-eight or thirty-one sober days, or any time in between). Instead, be a reference of information for curious friends, an outlier and trailblazer among your social circles, and, ultimately, someone who doesn't back down or give in to (sometimes excruciating) pressure!

Above all, don't take adverse reactions personally: Many people feel uncomfortable when their friends abandon drinking because this decision makes them ask themselves, "Should I do that, too?" For some, this question poses a challenge, which may be scary for them (and surely will shake up their habits if they choose to participate).

The lack of imbibing on your part can affect your friends' social plans, whether they state the obvious (they don't have a drinking buddy to go out with) or it's less apparent (they have a fear of missing out on your newfound hobbies). Remember to invite these pals to nondrinking adventures (even if they aren't giving up booze for the month) so they don't miss fun moments! Also, be sure to reiterate (unsarcastically) that you're not judging them for drinking—it's almost guaranteed they'll follow the same standard of politeness. If your friends aren't supporting your stance, it's not because they don't like you: It's because they're afraid of change. Honestly, they want you to have fun!

But if the conversation about this challenge turns awkward, and your friends, family, or acquaintances are relentlessly unsupportive about your Dry Jan (or another dry month), change the subject to a topic unrelated to booze. (Work! Family! Hobbies! The weather! Upcoming holidays and travel plans! The possibilities are endless . . . .) Chances are, unless you're a sommelier, bartender, distributor, salesperson, or spirits brand ambassador, you likely aren't constantly chatting about grape varietals, cocktail recipes, and beer trends. But, even if you are, those conversations have no bearing on how much or how little you're drinking this month. (Hint: The amount is zero. You are drinking nothing.) In any case, not imbibing is not an action that defines you. You're still you! And you can still debate, banter, and hold conversations about these topics and a million other subjects (just as you do in February and December, and so on).

You're still you!

. . . or Keep a Low Profile, If You Prefer

Grade school has passed, and so has playing passive-aggressive games (hopefully, at least). With that in mind, note that you don't *have* to participate in a conversation about why you don't want to drink in January (or any other month). If you're the type of person who doesn't need or want feedback, opt out. Don't tell people about your goals until you feel comfortable doing so or after you've passed the finish line.

The reality is that when you tell people about your dry-month journey, they might quiz you about it and even challenge your participation. So, if you're the type of person who gives in to peer pressure, stay mum! And when you're ready to talk about it, be strong!

Stand Firm

Don't give up the fight—and don't fight with your friends, either.
Instead of getting defensive or letting things escalate, calmly find out
what's really behind their seemingly aggressive questions. One year,
during Dry January, a friend became angry when I wouldn't drink with
her during her birthday party. After being bullied a bit, and feeling
super alienated, I thought to myself, "Well, I can leave now and risk
losing a friendship, or I can be an adult and figure out how to not only
coexist but to have fun!" We had a five-minute private chat and
resolved our issue. It turns out that when I announced I wasn't drinking, she had taken it as a sign that I didn't want to be there! (Well,
obviously, she was a little tipsy and misread my resistance to ordering
a cocktail.) She actually didn't care that I was choosing not to be
under the influence. What mattered to her was that I was part of the
group—having fun, hanging out, and not letting my thirty-one-day
commitment alienate me. As I ordered a soda water, I assured her that
my N.A. orders would go unnoticed. Fast-forward to the end of the
evening: We all had a great time. No one cared about my level (well,
lack) of consumption. She got drunk, her friends got wasted, and I
was completely buzz-free (and hangover-free the next morning).
Success!

Confidence, sans Cocktails

The bottom line: Go into Dry January with confidence and a positive
outlook. The community of individuals you typically imbibe with aren't
your enemies—they're curious individuals yearning for insight about a
challenge they haven't tried, or, more specifically, a concept they
haven't considered if you weren't taking it on. (Truthfully, it wouldn't

have even crossed their minds otherwise.) Appropriate responses to outsiders' comments might require further factual research. (So, when you're talking about the benefits of being dry or activities you've picked up in the absence of alcohol, see page 90 and page 106 as starting points and inspiration!) Remember: Regardless of which tough, specific, and loaded questions are being asked, when you prepare to deliver your thoughts in a self-assured manner, people will listen. They'll notice how empowered you feel, and they'll respect you for it.

And, after the initial round of interrogation, there's a good chance acquaintances will ask you for advice—in preparation for their own participation in the next year's Dry January or an upcoming Sober October. If they don't, as the next chapter shows, you'll see them the following month when your challenge is over.

The No-Cocktail Convo Cheat Sheet

Get ready for your friends, family, strangers, and every other soul you encounter during your sober month to suddenly pay attention to your nondrinking presence (or your absence) at the bar. Many will ask you about your dry commitment. Here's a cheat sheet to answering pesky "why" and "how" questions politely, creatively, and with confidence.

Q: WHY AREN'T YOU DRINKING?

A: I'm doing Dry [insert month here], and I've committed to being dry for [insert number here] days! Yay!

A: I'm not drinking tonight. I have an early morning tomorrow!

Q: DON'T YOU MISS DRINKING? IS IT HARD?

A: Yes, but one month is a short period of time if you really think about it . . . and I'm sticking to it. I'm still going out and seeing friends, just without drinking!

A: Not really. I've been doing other things instead, like going to the gym, catching up on movies, and going to more dinners with friends.

Q: WHY NOT HAVE ONE DRINK? ON ME.

A: I will, in [insert remaning number] days. [*Wink*.] I'll celebrate once the month is over.

A: Nah, not really in the mood. Plus I've already lasted [insert number here] days without beer, wine, and spirits. I can't give in now . . . but thank you!

Q: DO YOU FEEL DIFFERENT, NOT DRINKING?

A: I'm still having fun and going out . . . but I will say, not having a hangover the next morning feels so great.

A: Yeah! I sleep better at night. I have more energy, and I'm not spending a ton of money on booze!

Q: IS IT HARD TO DATE WHEN DRINKS AREN'T INVOLVED?

A: Isn't it hard to date, regardless? [*Laugh.*]

A: It's actually kind of liberating to find things to do besides going out for a drink! And you know, without a drink, you can tell right away whether you genuinely like that person or if it's the cocktails talking.

Q: WANT A BEER?

A: I'd love a cola.

A: No, thanks!

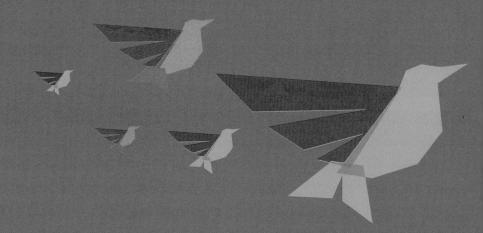

CHAPTER 8

When Birds of a Feather Don't Flock (to the Bar) Together

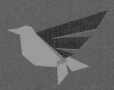

Remember that time you and your best friend from middle school promised to be in each other's lives forever (friendship bracelets, nicknames, inside jokes, and all) . . . and then high school rolled around and you both went your separate ways?

This may sound harsh, but the subject of this chapter is kind of like that. However, instead of music genres, extracurricular activities, and clothing choices dividing you and your teenage friends, the catalyst this time around, in adult life, is alcohol (more specifically, two teams: consuming and not consuming). These pages will address the effects on the company you keep, particularly your social circle, while you're undertaking Dry January or another block of time designated to staying dry.

All's Fair in Love and Wine

Point blank: Taking a firm no-drinking stance might be hard—not just for you, but also for your friends and acquaintances. Losing a key member of their drinking squad can feel devastating to them. Think of it this way: It's as if you're on a team at work and one person takes thirty-one days off—it's going to impact the group's productivity, or at least the group dynamic. (For example: Taylor from accounting isn't going to know what to do with your pay stub! Or, in this case, with whom to split the bar tab.) In essence, your drinking squad depends on you to have fun (and pay a portion of the bill).

If picking up potential soulmates (or bedmates) is something you and your friends bond over, Cupid might have to dust off his bow and arrow and get to work. Falling out of the pattern of wingman-ing (or wingwoman-ing) for your buds at the bar can change things up in the lives of others, not to mention your own life. You and your friends might not meet new love interests in their, or your, usual fashion. This isn't to say all of you can't do it alone, but the regular routine has been broken, and the vibe has inevitably shifted.

> **PRO TIP:** RATHER THAN POSTING UP AT THE BAR, OFFER TO WING(WO)MAN FOR FRIENDS AT PLACES WHERE BOOZE ISN'T THE HEADLINER. CONCERTS, SPORTING EVENTS, AND OTHER INTERACTIVE VENUES CAN INSPIRE GREAT CONVERSATION STARTERS AND INTRODUCTIONS TO NEW SIGNIFICANT OTHERS.

Friends also might take it personally if you choose to miss out on the emotional updates that often pour forth over drinks, should you decide it's too much of a temptation to go out. Dating dramas, family fights, and work dilemmas will have to be divulged over another (nonalcoholic) liquid and possibly in a different place. Having a weekly ritual of bonding over beers or wine won't suit sober-month standards. Instead of late nights out on weekends, chances are you'll be hitting the sack earlier, and cutting short the time you'd typically be hanging out and clinking cups or fancy wineglasses until the wee hours of the morning (because most businesses that aren't serving booze close at earlier times).

Enough of this friendship funeral! No one is breaking ties over melodramatic misunderstandings (and surely no bar fights are breaking out due to intoxication, that's for sure). As adults, you and your comrades will figure it out.

Make New Friends . . .

If your buddies insist on going to the bar without you, that's okay! Everyone's an adult here (and likely independent). Instead of boozing in your spare time, or watching them drink while you patiently sip soda water, take up different activities and invite new people to enter and actively participate in the things you want to do.

Branching out to other pastimes, new places, and social situations that go beyond boozing will open up spare time to connect with people you never knew existed. Think about it this way: Suddenly you have time to go to the gym at 7 p.m., and—guess what?—there are other people working out at that time. These are individuals you would have

If your buddies insist on going to the bar **without** you,

that's okay!

never spoken to or even seen before because your usual 7 p.m. slot was dedicated to drinking daiquiris. The same goes for other extracurricular activities: everything from Ping-Pong to playing pool.

While you may have gotten used to striking up new conversations with the help of liquid courage, approaching people and making friends without booze will be surprisingly easy—especially because there isn't a cerveza shield to hide behind.

1. **You and your potential new friend(s)** are in the same place at the same time, so you already have at least one common interest. (For example, you're both in a dog park: You either have a dog, or you like dogs.)

2. **Striking up a conversation** can be as simple as asking for help or a recommendation. (e.g., "What a great dog leash your puppy has. It's so stylish and functional. My dog's leash is getting old, and I was thinking of getting a new one. Where did you buy it?")

Case in point: You don't need whiskey to win people over and foster new relationships. This new-friend thing is a cinch.

. . . but Keep the Old

While you're breaking from your usual (drinking) routine, a dry month is the best time to seek out friends you've lost touch with over the years. Initiating conversations with former colleagues can be helpful for networking or just a friendly nonwork-related catch-up. Maybe it's time to bury the hatchet or even restart things with an ex-girlfriend/ boyfriend/person (tread lightly, depending on the circumstances). Specifically, if your former fling—or fiancé(e), or anything in between— ended things citing booze being a factor in finishing the relationship, a dry month could be a great time to revisit this important person and reconnect on a safe and even playing field. The commitment to not drink for a designated period of time might have a serious impact on your former relationship (or perhaps none at all, but it's worth exploring). As far as nonromantic friendships go: If you've bonded with people in your past over something besides booze, see if you can pick up where you left off. Even if you were on the same rec basketball team in elementary school, why not extend an invite to watch a sports game on TV or in person? Or get active, and find a basketball court where you can shoot hoops.

One Is Silver and the Other's Gold
(. . . and Neither of Them Is Tequila)

Drinking may be one of the ties that bind some of your friendships—which isn't necessarily a bad thing. But you might want to explore other ways to get together with friends and, ultimately, share experiences outside the influence of alcohol. Even if your close circle of friends is drinking through January, you can also hang with them when they aren't imbibing. While your go-to spots may be designated areas for getting bombed, that doesn't mean that you haven't spent time with them elsewhere in the past. (Right?) And, even if you haven't, you can start now.

Once you remove alcohol from your friendships, you may also notice that you bond with people differently—and for the better! Rather than scream-talking nonsense, at one another in a loud and crowded bar, you can have the same conversations (or even better, deeper chats) in a quiet cafe, from across a dinner table, in a coffee shop, or even at home. The change of scenery might inspire newfound respect, dialogue, and topics of conversation. After all, there's a different attitude in the atmosphere when alcohol isn't playing a leading role. For example, taking shots and belting out the lyrics to an old pop song at a dive bar is super fun, but the whiskey-filled atmosphere isn't likely going to lead to a heartfelt conversation about family. When alcohol is involved, late nights might end with a drunk sob and an ugly cry (with or without the involvement of pop ballads).

PRO TIP: IF YOU REALLY WANT TO SING SOMETHING IN PUBLIC, HIT UP A KARAOKE BAR AND LEAVE THE BOOZE BEHIND. IF SINGING TO AN AUDIENCE WITHOUT A BUZZ SOUNDS TERRIFYING, TAKE YOUR SING-ALONG SKILLS INTO THE COMFORT OF YOUR HOME WITH A HAIRBRUSH AS YOUR MIC AND YOUTUBE AS YOUR LYRICS GUIDE.

Although people often bond over drinking, the truth is that by not imbibing, you can keep a steady focus on your friend sharing his or her deep, dark, and personal secrets. Without the influence of alcohol, your attention span, concentration, and memory just function better.

You'll be able to recall these sacred stories the next day in so much more detail when vodka isn't involved.

When You Come Back Around

Admittedly, your time off from cocktails may also result in time away from the local dive bar, and, furthermore, translate into a brief hiatus from the other eleven months of your booze-influenced social life. So, when it's time to end your dry spell (whether that's on the first day of a new month, or any time after . . . or not at all—hey, keep going for as long as you'd like!), there's a good chance you'll return to your old stomping grounds and see your (not-so-) long-lost friends. Note that getting reacquainted with buddies can take more than just seconds. If you haven't seen a person or group of people in one month, you'll naturally have a lot of catching up to do.

If you choose to participate in Dry Jan, specifically, the same questions that you dealt with in early January, such as "Why partici-pate in Dry January?" and "How do you feel?" and "Do you miss drinking?" will likely come up when your month is completed. And, by now, you'll be a pro at answering these queries with confidence. (Not to mention you'll be able to describe the amazing benefits from a first-person perspective.)

Beyond reconnecting with familiar faces, and sharing what you've been doing when you haven't been drinking, now is a fitting time—as your reunions are taking place—to reflect on how these people contribute to your life as a whole (if at all).

- **Did you miss** seeing them at the bar?
- **Did you forget,** or not care, that they were absent from your life?
- **Do you feel** relieved or sad, that you missed out on drinking-induced shenanigans?
- **Does their presence** bring you joy when you see them, or not so much?

Like many other facets of this month-long challenge, reacquainting yourself with these comrades will be an adjustment.

But it isn't just you who is impacted by your dry days. The people you typically surround yourself with will have to adapt, change their ways, or simply follow suit (and maybe not drink . . . as much, or at all, with you).

Don't be surprised if they admit they missed you, that they cut down on cocktails as well (because they didn't have a drinking buddy), or they just stopped going out completely without your company!

Or, your challenge might not change your personal relationships at all. Seriously. You might keep the same schedule, routine, friends, and after-hours lifestyle that you did the day before your challenge started (minus the booze). If so, and it's working for you: Congrats! That's great! If not, keep reading.

How to Make Friends without the Influence of Alcohol

In grade school, recruiting a new BFF was as easy as sharing the red crayon in art class. As an adult, sometimes these exchanges can be a little bit more difficult—or at least less common. (After all, how often are you coloring at work, or in your spare time?) Have no fear, the ability to reconnect with old friends, meet people, and form friendships doesn't have to entail communal craft supplies or inebriation. To start, here are some prompts that will help you spark conversations with people from your past, present, and future.

WITH A FORMER COWORKER . . .

"I know it's been a bit since you/I left the company, but I'd love to pick your brain about some work stuff if you're free sometime this month."

WITH A CHILDHOOD BEST FRIEND . . .

"Remember that time we snuck into an R-rated movie when we were in middle school? I think we're past that, but I saw the sequel is finally coming out this weekend. Should we go?"

WITH AN
EX . . .

"Hi, hope you're doing well. Would love to make time for tea or a snack this week and catch up!"

WITH A
NEW PERSON AT THE GYM . . .

"Have you taken the cardio class here? It looks challenging! I'm up to try it if you are."

WITH A
POTENTIAL FRIEND AT THE DOG PARK, OR A FELLOW DOG-WALKER ON THE SIDEWALK . . .

"Your dog is so cute! What's his or her name?"

WITH A
NEIGHBOR YOU ALWAYS RUN INTO BUT NEVER MAKE TIME FOR . . .

"Have you checked out the new cafe in our neighborhood? Let's grab a coffee or a bite and hang out!"

WITH
ANYONE ELSE . . .

"Hi. How are you?"

CHAPTER 9

Sober Month Support Squad

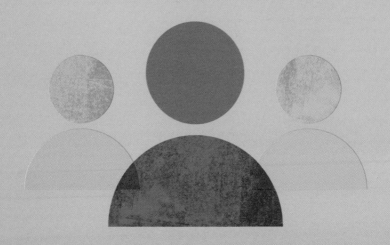

For many dry-month participants, a parent or sibling could be more supportive than, say, your circle of party buddies from college. (But who knows! Maybe Grandma is the reigning keg-stand champ and your family gets competitive during tailgates. No judgment here.) Feedback from friends, relatives, and strangers about your temporary lifestyle change may be thrown in your face on Day One or creep up on you during Week Two—or even appear when you first mention your commitment, perhaps in December before your Dry January begins.

Fret not: There are many ways to request support from people near and dear to you—and encourage fellow participants, too. And note that even if people are picking on you, nagging you to join in on boozing, or making you feel like you're missing out, there's sure to be some admiration in the mix, too.

How to Ask for a Shot of Support

Determine how to utilize your squad to best accomplish your goals. Do you want someone checking in with you daily? Weekly? Or not at all? Do you prefer to rally all of your fellow challengers in group chats or activities, or speak to and see people one at a time? Beyond hangtime with dry-buddies, you might want to think through real-life scenarios and how to approach them. If you're going to brunch with a friend who orders bottomless drinks (or having dinner at home with your significant other, who pops open a bottle of wine), ask him or her to consider having a meal with you without an imbibing component. Of course, your friend (or bae) is allowed to decline, but that's one of the little things you can request from the people around you to make yourself more comfortable. After all, if you don't ask, you won't receive!

It's equally imperative to pay it forward (read: treat others how you want to be treated, and in this case, instill confidence in fellow participants). Giving verbal encouragement comes naturally to some people, but it's totally reasonable (and commendable) to need and show positive reinforcement in other ways, like arranging N.A. activities or gifting N.A. beverages. Just like love languages, everyone shows kindness and empathy differently (and admit it, you do, too).

If you're part of a Sober Month Support Squad yourself: In order to empower your favorite dry sister or mister, ask her or him how you can help. Inquire about favorite things to do (outside of bars) and see what her or his plans are for that range of dates. Gauge your comrade's interest in teaming up for group or one-on-one dinners, coffee meetups, or other hangouts—see how you can encourage success (without overstepping boundaries and getting annoying).

Role Models (No Bottles): Set the Tone

You're likely not the only person around who is committing to a booze-free month, so be a champion for fellow partakers. Strength in numbers! And, if you don't succeed this time (or you choose not to participate in future years), you can still cheer on your dry friends.

Share these few pointers with your still-boozing buddies—everyone can benefit from knowing a few easy tips to making nonimbibers feel at ease.

1. **Show respect and compassion** by not guilting abstainers into drinking, such as ordering them alcoholic beverages they don't want or inviting them into situations where drinking will be strongly encouraged.
2. **Plan social activities** that can be held in places other than bars or clubs.
3. **Show consideration and sensitivity** by asking if the abstaining person (or people) feels comfortable in booze-heavy situations.

No-Alcohol Accountability

Having a friend, or at least an acquaintance, who is a fellow dry-month participant to check in with on a regular basis (weekly, daily, hourly—whatever you need) can be a kind reminder that you're not alone in your journey. Touching base isn't a requirement (by any means) or bound to a set schedule. It can be as casual as texting "hello," followed by a string of emojis, or it can be a full deep-dive convo via phone or video chat. The frequency and depth of these conversations are guided by (who else!) you.

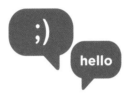

Once you find your no-cocktail comrade, or crew, you'll have a partner (or pact pack) who can relate and understand (at least some of) what you're going through.

Take advantage of the fact that, during your absence from the bar, you might notice more money in the bank (and your dry friends will likely see the same savings, too). Alongside your Sober Month Support Squad, spend that extra cash having dinner together at fancy dinners (or over froyo) to celebrate weekly. During these regularly scheduled gatherings, you can catch up on highs and lows, review how you're feeling, and discuss changes to your personal and professional lives. This gives everyone an opportunity to stay social yet resist the temptation of a less-reassuring atmosphere (like a club or dive bar).

Potential topics during these meetups or group chats via text message can include the difficulty and/or ease of declining a drink, awkward moments when responding to temptation, and the benefits of not imbibing (". . . OMG my skin is soooo clear!"). Even if you and your Sober Month Support Squad don't have very much else in common (e.g., job, age, gender, recreational interests, a mortgage), abstaining from booze is a bond-forming commitment that breaks through a lot of social, political, occupational, and even economic barriers.

Another benefit of having an understanding Sober Month Support Squad is learning from them. Your nonimbibing buddy (or buddies) will have tips, suggestions, and ideas for alternative activities that will help breeze through the first month (or any month) of the year without guzzling wine after a stressful day (or even a super successful one). You, too, will influence them in a positive manner, offering your own guidance, assistance, and ears when they are in need of help.

PRO TIP: EVEN A SIMPLE ACTION LIKE TEXTING A PHOTO OF SELTZER WATER TO A FRIEND OR TO THE GROUP CHAT CAN ACT AS A SUBTLE REMINDER THAT IT'S IMPORTANT TO STICK IT OUT, AND THAT YOU'RE WITH THEM IN SPIRIT (EVEN WITHOUT SPIRITS).

Social Media Status: #DryAF

Stay hush-hush, or announce your challenge from the rooftops with a megaphone. Preach about your challenge as much you want on the Internet and other phone apps that condone sharing your personal updates. Verified influencer or not, many people announce their status proudly via social media—and who knows? Maybe you'll start a new category of social media influencer. On another note: don't let strangers from the web convince you not to partake in or succeed at a dry challenge—especially if you didn't ask for their opinion in the first place. Sometimes dry months can be challenging, and slip-ups can happen. This is just another way of being transparent on the Internet (These folks may just need a little encouragement!) Go on: Interact! Like, double-tap and respond with your well wishes!

Among your Sober Month Support Squad, showcase your creativity using personalized hashtags. These can allude to the abstaining crew in your area using area codes, like #dryjan305 (for residents of Miami, Florida), or counting down the days #72hoursintodryjan (for an hour-by-hour update, with new hashtags weekly, daily—or hourly if you dare) or inside jokes like #dryjanbet2win. You can even schedule a brainstorming session to collaborate. And don't feel as though you're limited to just one or two hashtags—the possibilities are endless!

STAY HUSH-HUSH **X**

ANNOUNCE YOUR
CHALLENGE FROM
THE ROOFTOPS

SHARE YOUR
PERSONAL UPDATES
(OR CHANGE YOUR
STATUS)

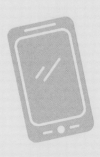

Reaching out to support a stranger isn't a bad idea either, as long as you're not a creep (read: Please be mindful and respectful of boundaries . . . you know, keep it G-rated and don't stalk people. Okay?). It's cool to support participants and comment on posts in Dry January Facebook groups, pages, and message boards—the same goes for Instagram and Twitter. On Reddit, join the conversation and add to all kinds of topic threads by answering relevant questions, extending advice, and bonding over common experiences associated with an alcohol-free month.

In the same way you're instilling others with confidence about their dry-month journeys on the web, you, too, can ask for help on the Internet! Get real on your own handles within your favorite social media platforms and via dry-month message boards, and share if you're having a hard time. Asking for advice and words of encouragement isn't just okay, it's great! You'll get the feedback you're looking for and feel empowered in real time.

INTO THE AIRWAVES

To consume advice (without the reaction of others), Alcohol Change UK delivers a podcast, too, right to your phone (or computer) if you need a verbal reminder as to why you're making a commitment to this (not-so-long-but-seemingly-long) period of time. On the Try Dry Podcast, which can be accessed through the Alcohol Change UK website, they cover the ups and downs, lifestyle changes, and, naturally, the benefits of nixing booze for a month.

And, while podcasts focused on booze, drinking, bartending, and everything spirits-related exist, there are plenty of chatty individuals who don't talk about imbibing on their shows. Most hosts talk regularly about all other subjects ranging from dating and sports and weddings to entrepreneurship and health and more. By listening to new topics (especially those that don't concern your time at the bar), you may even take up another hobby or interest that you hadn't thought about otherwise.

Imitation Is the Sincerest Form of Flattery

Much like that time you bought a killer pair of jeans and your best friend couldn't help but follow your lead and buy them, too, you may also notice that your dry month (like your immaculate fashion sense) rubs off on others. Once you declare you're not drinking for a few weeks, friends and family may join you on the month-long journey, or at least cut down on their intake. Together, you can strategize other activities and talk about the struggles (or ease) and day-to-day (love/hate) feelings about keeping dry—even if they aren't fully committed to the full month or weren't initially interested in participating. And, if you want to make things really interesting, propose a friendly bet with a buddy (or a few bets with a handful of friends).

Place a No-Booze Bet

Perhaps all of the amazing benefits of a dry month don't appeal to you (for whatever reason), but winning is something you love to do! A bet—either a friendly wager or one with some real prizes at stake—might light a fire inside and encourage you to push through tough times in order to meet your booze-free goal.

Looking forward to redeeming prizes—or the thought of paying up (or paying forward something you don't want to do) if you lose—can be motivating factors. For instance, if you're excited for your friend to buy you a new pair of shoes (if you win), keep reminding yourself that those pricey sneakers are worth it (and how good they will look with the jeans you already own)! Alternatively, if you really, really don't want to babysit your friend's kid or cat (if they win), then remember how you hate cleaning up after that child (or fur child). Whatever your incentives are, stick it out! You can do this!

After choosing your competitors, collectively decide what the champions will obtain after completing a designated time frame without any wine, beer, or spirits. Winners are bestowed bragging rights (naturally), but maybe their drinks or dinner are paid for by the Damp Camp (participants who tried but did not succeed) by the time a new month rolls around. (More on a Demi-Sec—aka Medium Dry—month on page 202). Perhaps the victors are treated to a movie of their choice, a workout class they've been wanting to try, or an adventure that does not involve alcohol.

friends who **don't** drink together . . . **won't** be hungover in the morning.

Whatever the parameters, three components are definite: no drinking, no cheating, and no sabotaging the other participants!

Celebrate Your Accomplishments Together

Every day marks a new mile marker for you and your no-cocktails crew, so it's important to acknowledge that each and every booze-free week is a step in the right direction. You've helped each other not mess it all up—and maybe, if someone has, you've helped them restart. (Check page 196 for some ideas!)

When the month winds down (read: is officially over—and not a day before), get together with the ones who got you through the tough times (and who you went to bat for, as well)! Share a drink, or go on and celebrate with an N.A. beverage. It's your night (or day)!

After all, the friends who don't drink together . . . will not be hungover in the morning. And that goes for singles who are dating and established couples, too.

SIDE NOTE: You don't need nondrinking buddies to gamble. You can make a bet with your friends who are drinking during the month, or bet against yourself. If you win, treat yourself to those super-comfy sneakers you've been eyeing, or that trip to Australia you can't stop dreaming about. If you lose, hold yourself accountable: Extend your dry days for an extra few days past the finish line. Prizes are motivating, but the big win is making it to the end, as you'll soon find out! This element will keep you honest and motivated (and competitive) in the meantime.

Feeling Lucky?

Take bets to the next level with your Sober Month Support Squad
and hold each other accountable! You can also wager with
friends (nondrinkers and drinkers alike) . . . or place a personal
bet with yourself!

List who you're betting against and what the winners receive
upon succeeding, as well as what the fallen Sober Month Support
Squad members (aka "Honorable Mentions") must do/give upon
slipping up.

EXAMPLE

A BET WITH: Alejandro

WINNER WINS: A meal at any restaurant in New York City.

HONORABLE MENTIONS MUST: Pay for said meal.

IF WE BOTH WIN: We will split a bottle of Champagne in celebration
over dinner. We will split the bill at the restaurant.

IF WE BOTH LOSE: No fancy feasting. No Champagne.

BET 1

A BET WITH:

WINNER WINS:

HONORABLE MENTIONS MUST:

IF WE BOTH/ALL WIN:

IF WE BOTH/ALL LOSE:

BET 2

A BET WITH:

WINNER WINS:

HONORABLE MENTIONS MUST:

IF WE BOTH/ALL WIN:

IF WE BOTH/ALL LOSE:

BET 3

A BET WITH:

WINNER WINS:

HONORABLE MENTIONS MUST:

IF WE BOTH/ALL WIN:

IF WE BOTH/ALL LOSE:

CHAPTER 10

D(N)UI—Dating (Not) Under the Influence

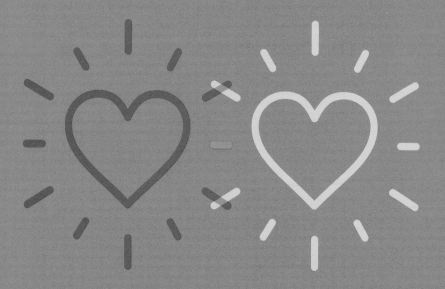

Here's a fun chapter! The dating world is already chock-full of confusing rules, preferences (transparently: requirements), and expectations, so why not add one more to the mix . . . right?

"Going for a drink" is the norm for dating, especially when you're first getting to know someone—but not when you're doing a dry month! Have no fear: You can still have fun, get to know someone, and carry on as your amazing, flirty, desirable self. The only difference is there is no alcohol involved, which, in turn, might inspire some other changes to your regularly scheduled programming.

Date + Flirting – Alcohol = Still a Date

Extracting alcohol from the dating-game equation impacts much more than where you go on said date. (How often are adults' first dates spent innocently sipping milkshakes at the diner or waiting in line at an ice cream scoop shop? Answer: While it sounds adorable, the truth is: Not so frequently.) Boozing also affects how you feel (while drinking and in the hours/day after), what you say (while intoxicated and during a hangover), and how you act (inhibitions = gone, or at least more liberal), among other intimate elements (from personal boundaries to the bedroom).

Cocktails calm nerves and lubricate conversations, but they are not a prereq for a good time and/or a successful date. (PSA: You can still flirt and engage in meaningful conversations without an IPA.) By eliminating the glossy booze screen, there is no flirtatious, mysterious veil to hide behind. Dating during a dry month may sound as relaxing as plunging naked into the Antarctic Ocean—but unlike the frigid water temperature, which you're unlikely to acclimate to, you will, in fact, adapt to meeting potential love interests without wine and other alcoholic beverages. Yes, the absence of drinks might inspire moments of silence between sips of water, but you'll find ways to fill the gaps with great conversation. And if you don't, perhaps this person isn't the one for you. Rest assured, there are major upsides to saying "see you later" to lager.

A Round of Drinks vs. Reality

"Beer goggles" is the term for when you drink, and, as a result, think people are more attractive than they are in reality. In other words, the alcohol is messing with your vision. Yes, this is a real thing (free with the purchase of too many drinks). Booze not only helps people cover up who they are but also throws off one's perception of another person's true character. Whether you order a Mind Eraser cocktail or you're slowly consuming cervezas, alcohol clouds your judgment, slows your reaction time, and prompts you to jump to conclusions about the integrity of the other imbiber across the table from you. All in all, what you see is not what you (really) get. Starting off a relationship with such an inaccurate perception can be a problem. On one hand, you might think someone is infinitely better and more awesome than he or she really is, when in reality, this person is a lowlife covering up terrible, undesirable qualities. On the other hand, you might risk losing out on an opportunity to get to know someone for who he or she truly is because the beer in your hand has led you to believe this person is not a match (when the truth is, he or she is perfectly complementary to your personality and exactly the kind of person you're looking to date . . . or marry)!

Imbibing also impacts how you interact with your date and how your date interacts with you. When tipsiness takes charge, people tend to flirt more overtly, act more aggressively, have a compromised attention span, and the like. Alcohol prompts a range of internal effects, too: from subduing anxieties you have about behaviors (that would otherwise stand out as red flags) to causing an artificially elevated mood (when in real life, not under the influence, you would actually be bored out of your mind and desperate to retreat ASAP). When time is spent with an incompatible person, sans a shared margarita pitcher, you'll likely realize sooner that the two of you are not on the same level spiritually, emotionally, or otherwise. These judgments matter because they're formed as you're building the foundation with a potential S.O., a seasonal fling, a fun friend with (or without) benefits, or even your future spouse!

Picking Up Dates (Rather Than the Tab)

If you're single (and looking . . . and maybe your New Year's resolution involves meeting a new love), Dry January will influence how you meet people (romantically or otherwise). The places you'll get hit on, and the locations in which you pursue a potential special someone, will shift away from drinking-centric events like happy hours and tailgates. In addition, with more nondrinking activities making up your day-to-day schedule, you'll be exposed to a new pool of people, and you're likely to meet different individuals with similar interests to yours. It'll be no surprise, too, that the (dry) men and women you meet face-to-face during an alcohol-free month will be comfortable participating in things that don't involve booze during the rest of the year. Meeting someone who isn't under the influence (and being attracted to this person without the support of beer, wine, and spirits) is most definitely a positive realization: When you've consumed 0 percent alcohol, you know your attraction is 100 percent unsullied. The same can be said for the person who likes you—it's a win-win: The booze isn't talking; your feelings are organically coming from the heart!

APPS-TAINING FROM ALCOHOL

When swiping right and left for love on popular dating apps, build a profile with information and photos that truly represent your amazing, one-of-a-kind self—especially when you've committed to a booze-free month. Whether you're looking for your soulmate, a relationship, a date, or a one-night thing, it's okay to state loud and proud that temporarily giving up alcohol (and everything that entails) is high priority (e.g., "Hi! My name is Jaime. I'm not drinking this month, but I'd love to get together for dinner or coffee this week."). Of course, you have the option of not mentioning it at all—but because it's a month-long commitment and part of your lifestyle for a handful of weeks, the topic will arise soon enough.

NO-WINE WARNING

How far along in the month you are will play into your decision to disclose your commitment, whether it's displayed on your main profile or through private chats.

- **During the first half of the month,** openness is the best (and most attractive) policy: Explain to a possible date that you won't be drinking but it's not a forever thing.
- **In the second half of the month,** as you near the finish, you may want to mention your dry challenge if you're planning a romantic rendezvous before the end of the month—to be fully transparent and also to give your date a heads-up about what to expect during your time together. There are several reasons: Honesty can be surprising—and impressive—on a first date. It's also good to be clear about your booze-free commitment, because the other person might be expecting liquid courage to help boost his or her confidence. Telling your date about your endeavor ahead of time will also avoid potentially giving the wrong impression (like the notion that you are sick and avoiding mixing medication with booze—no one wants to catch a cold!). Also, here's something new and different to talk about!
- **Finally,** if you're chatting up a storm with a girl or guy (whom you've never met before) during the tail end of your challenge, and making plans for the upcoming weeks (when you'll be drinking again), it might not impact your date night at all. The choice is yours!

Pour Your Heart Out

As you're taking inventory of how alcohol influences your day-to-day friendships and relationships with family, coworkers, and acquaintances, romantic relationships will fall into the same two categories: what's working vs. what isn't. A dry month is the best time to weed through the frogs and find your prince(ss)—or whatever kind of fairy-tale, magical happy ending that best suits you (shining armor and wine chalice not included).

If you're already in a relationship, and if date night routinely involves getting hammered, a dry month will allow you to see how you feel about your girlfriend, boyfriend, fiancé(e), husband, wife, or

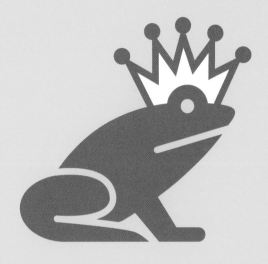

WEED THROUGH THE FROGS

partner when you aren't actively sloshed. Alcohol-free date nights can help you feel more connected and stronger as a couple, while facilitating chatting—and meaningful dialogue—about a wider range of topics. Comparing this experience with your typical nights out (or nights in) can help the two of you figure out alternative activities and shared interests to continue to bond over, especially if you decide it's time for the tequila train to make its final stop.

If you find that booze is the glue holding you together, and you're okay with that: Cool. No judgment. And if the reality is you don't have as much in common, maybe it's time to cut ties. This can be heart-breaking . . . or liberating, depending on whether your glass is half empty or half full (of club soda). While letting go of a person who chooses beer over his or her significant other can be devastating, imagine committing to spending years with this partner only to find out that you only really tolerate each other when you're sharing a bottle of wine. (Yikes!)

Designated Dater

Participating in dry months is actually a turn-on! For one: You're displaying you can commit to something (and probably someone . . . swoon!) and follow through with the promises you make. Two: You're not going to get sloppy drunk on a date (and make an idiot of yourself in public). Three: Your pledge demonstrates responsibility, honesty, self-control, and accountability. (Okay, that last was four reasons in one but really, who wants an irresponsible, dishonest, and immature other half? No thanks. Like close friends, the best partners are the ones you can count on, who are truthful, and who show up when you need them the most.)

Last: You don't rely on alcohol to have fun, *and* you get creative on dates . . . Need we say more? (When you're in an official relationship by Valentine's Day and married by March, be sure to include a wedding toast about not drinking!)

On the first, second, or third dates (or in conversations leading up to meeting up), explaining the parameters of your challenge doesn't have to be a long, drawn-out Q&A. It can be as simple as saying or texting, "I have something fun in mind: [insert activity here]. I'm doing Dry Jan and won't be drinking until February 1, but you're welcome to order a drink, if you'd like!" If your date isn't aware of the dry month trend, now would be a great time to teach them about it! Your date might be interested in joining in, or not at all, or doing something in between, like drinking when he or she isn't around you but keeping dry in your presence out of respect and support.

No-Drink Date Ideas

When drinking becomes synonymous with dating, there's little to no creativity involved. While there are many upsides to not drinking and dating, a big one is a change of scenery and routine! Picking a place to meet and ordering a beverage (no matter the destination, cocktail menu, or the person sitting across from you) can become a mundane, boring chore. And who wants that? Dry dates can get you out of your comfort zone, and also out on the town—in a different capacity. To begin with, suggesting a lounge or bar to meet up is a fine choice (even without ordering booze), but why not try a place where alcohol isn't the main event? Given the choice, most would pick exciting, fun get-togethers (or at least attention-grabbing outings) with personality rather than predictable ones. (This applies to all kinds of dating, friendships, and hangouts—unless you want to live the same days and dates over and over again . . . in which case, disregard any invitations for new, cool experiences and keep that tired, well-seasoned regimen going strong.)

No "Drink Minimum" Dates

While drinking dictates many romantic get-togethers, there are tons of fun, interactive date ideas that don't require a drink minimum, bottle service, or (on most occasions) an ID for proof of age. These activities are also much easier to do (gracefully) when you aren't buzzed.

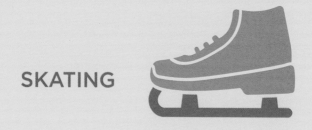

SKATING

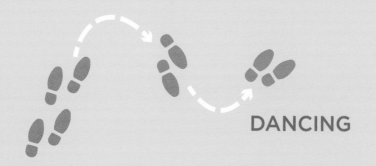

DANCING

GO-KARTS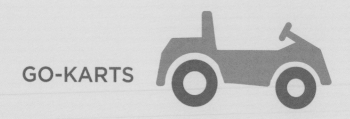

ICE SKATING AND ROLLER-SKATING

Gliding around a rink can facilitate conversation, bonding, and trust (especially when you can help each other not fall down)! Additionally, these are great spots for icebreaker conversations (pun intended) including people-watching those super-serious competition skaters and cute little kids with helicopter parents, in addition to pointing out funky outfits worn by fellow attendees. (And yes, you, too, can totally rock that pink tutu—don't let anyone tell you otherwise!)

DANCING

A dance lesson is another way to get closer to your date without yelling sloppily into each other's ears. Look into ballroom, salsa, tango, swing, and other types of dancing taught in private lessons or in groups at studios—or, for something more modern, hip-hop and breakdancing classes, too. Note: Spinning your partner is often par for the course (but not in a bad, drank-too-much, need-to-vomit kind of way).

If you're both really into music (and a club scene) but aren't the dancing types, some cities have DJ classes that anyone at any level can attend!

GO-KARTS

Adrenaline junkies can unite behind the wheel on a track. Just like driving a real car, go-kart racing and drinking do not mix, so the perfect time to take advantage of your desire to push the pedal to the metal—you speed demon, you—is when alcohol is zero part of the equation. Take your cutie on a ride (some racing tracks have two-seat karts) or face off and race to the finish! In this case, there's a clear reason for not imbibing before or during your date. (While the pace of your relationships should only be determined by you and your significant other, this activity is definitely best for those who like to move fast behind the wheel.)

Sex without Beer Goggles

Keeping dry does not mean the rest of your activities (and life) have to be G-rated (in case this wasn't obvious: being dry and being celibate are not one and the same). Not drinking will affect your sex life—but probably not how you might predict. Whether you hook up more or less, the precautions, the physical nuts and bolts of sex, and how you experience it will change.

Case in point: When you and your partner are abstaining from alcohol, there is zero chance of alcohol-inspired hookups or blurred lines relating to alcohol consumption. This is important when you consider the dangers of alcohol-related date rape and sexual assault.

On the most basic level, consuming alcohol dulls the senses and hinders sexual experiences (read: Some organs, um, don't function as they should). Alcohol is a depressant, and for men, it can sedate their member, and, well, its ability to perform. There is not an exact number of drinks or a particular type of spirit that discourages an erection—it's different for everyone. For women, it can dehydrate lady parts and cause discomfort and even pain! But without alcohol, there is zero chance that beer (or any alcoholic beverage) will get in the way of consensual hookups.

Without booze, you're both more aware of the need to use protection—and in control. Alcohol consumption does not affect the functioning of IUDs, the pill, the patch, and other forms of birth control when these are used correctly, according to Planned Parenthood. However, many studies show that under the influence of alcohol, people are less inclined to use condoms correctly, resulting in the contraction of STDs and STIs and unplanned pregnancies.

Respecting the No-Rum, No-Rye Regimen

It should be noted: Just because you're dry doesn't mean the cute guy or girl sitting across the table from you will skip out on sipping sangria, too. Which is totally okay. Keep in mind, less than a month ago you were drinking, and you'll probably drink again!

The bottom line: Dates are often a time to analyze actions to see if the person you're courting is a fit. And your date is definitely judging you, too. (Relax, it's natural!) During these hangouts, you can gauge how your date feels about your commitment and if this person acknowledges and respects your boundaries. Is he or she supportive of your decision? Does your date feel comfortable ordering a drink and consuming it solo? Or does he or she (try to) pressure you to order a cocktail . . . or order a beer on your behalf? Does your date choose to remain dry for the duration of your get-together, or does he or she get wasted in protest? Is your date open to making plans that don't revolve around alcohol? You'll gather the answers to these questions pretty quickly. The outcome will reveal whether your values and your date's align (at least when it comes to imbibing).

The good news is if you feel like it's a match, you'll see this person again. And if it's not, spend no more time thinking about it. You will have saved yourself from a (figuratively speaking) wasted night. And ponder the fact that you might have extended this relationship far past its expiration under false pretenses! The dry dating rule book (quick refresher: one rule—no booze) wins again!

And if you're not in the dating scene right now, you can still dress up, celebrate life, and do things that make you the happiest, solo. Heck, you can even throw a party for yourself (friends and attendees optional)!

Check, Please!

Dry dating isn't limited to boring ideas—it's all about engaging activities and creative date spots. Use this "choose your own adventure" questionnaire to inspire out-of-the-box and interactive evenings that don't revolve around drinking!

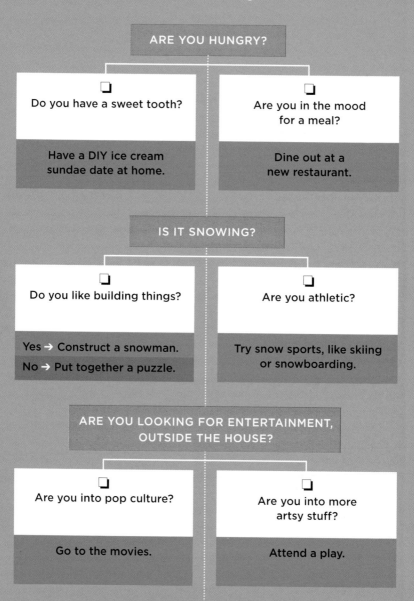

ARE YOU HUNGRY?

☐ Do you have a sweet tooth?

Have a DIY ice cream sundae date at home.

☐ Are you in the mood for a meal?

Dine out at a new restaurant.

IS IT SNOWING?

☐ Do you like building things?

Yes → Construct a snowman.
No → Put together a puzzle.

☐ Are you athletic?

Try snow sports, like skiing or snowboarding.

ARE YOU LOOKING FOR ENTERTAINMENT, OUTSIDE THE HOUSE?

☐ Are you into pop culture?

Go to the movies.

☐ Are you into more artsy stuff?

Attend a play.

FEELING MUSICAL?

❏
Do you want to listen to other people play instruments or dance?

Rock out at a concert.

❏
Would you prefer to play your own music?

Learn something new together, like how to DJ.

HAVE A KNACK FOR SPORTS?

❏
Do you want to relax and watch other people play?

Attend a sports game and cheer on your favorite teams together (or in rivalry).

❏
Looking to get your sweat on?

Find a basketball court or batting cages.

NEED SOME MORE SPEED?

❏
Want to feel tires on the street?

Race go-karts—together in one vehicle, or side by side in two.

❏
Just want to get behind any wheel?

Go to an arcade and race virtually!

COMPETITIVE BY NATURE?

❏
Want to stay in?

Host a game night to challenge each other's minds and strategy skills.

❏
Want to go out?

Find a trivia night focused on entertainment or other topics of mutual interest.

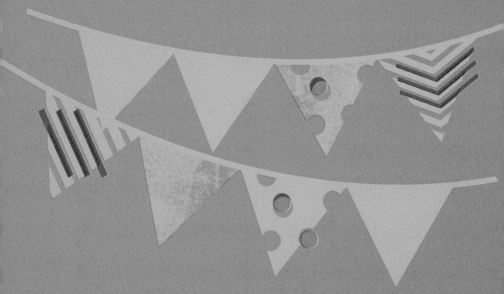

CHAPTER 11

Throw
an N.A.
Shindig

It's time to take a moment (and maybe a few hours, with friends in tow) to celebrate, in the midst of your booze-free regimen, how far you've come since Day One (and, yes, you can totally throw a shindig on Day Two if it suits you). Even if you're not chugging beers or going shot-for-shot (or respectfully sipping a cocktail or a glass of Pinot Noir), you can still party!

Wherever you are on your voyage, you've likely replaced cocktails, drinking-related activities, and social engagements at bars and nightclubs with nonalcoholic beverages, nonimbibing plans, and drink-free thingies. But spending a night out (or in) without booze can be as festive and social as any other date during any other month of the year. Sometimes you just need a little inspiration . . .

A No-Booze Flashback Birthday Bonanza

If you're celebrating another trip around the sun during your dry month, happy [insert age here] birthday! You knew you could have used your big day as an alibi and a reason to drink whatever alcoholic beverage your heart desired, but look at you—throwing an alcohol-free fiesta instead! (Applause ensues.)

First and foremost: It's your day! Plan your birthday the way you envision it! Grab dinner with a small (or large) group of friends and leave the prep and execution to the pros. Or opt for a night out (without mezcal) or an activity like b-day bowling. Or even go retro, with a party that is reminiscent of at-home childhood commemorations of yesteryear. Instead of beer, serve soda pop or a nonalcoholic punch (you know, the things you'd drink at youth celebrations). During your throwback birthday, play games like pin the tail on the donkey and smash a piñata (two contests you'll undoubtedly feel safer doing without the consumption of alcohol—for your own sake *and* the sake of your guests). Change up drinking-inspired games, like Water Pong (instead of Beer Pong) and Flipcup (without booze), among other mini-tournaments.

Another perk to having a party that doesn't revolve around drinking: Getting home safely isn't a concern, because those who are driving definitely won't be imbibing during your soiree. And, rather than having your guests part ways with the drunken munchies (and unhappy hangovers the next day), sweeten the rest of their week with thoughtful favors like home-baked (or store-bought) cookies (or candy from the piñata).

Booze-Free Bake-Off

Rather than consuming sugary drinks, hone in on your cravings in a hands-on way! Organize and host a showcase of N.A. baked goods (with or without an event entry fee). Challenge your friends to put on their thinking caps (and chef hats and aprons, too, if they so fancy . . . read: no drinking pants, please!). See page 166 for some fun recipes!

Establish some ground rules:
- Inform participants that they are free to create any kind of baked good, including bread, cookies, brownies, tarts, cakes, cupcakes, pies, pastries, donuts, and beyond!
- These delicacies should be made to abide by all participating eaters' dietary restrictions (e.g., gluten-free, dairy-free, nut-free, and so on).
- All bake-off items must (without a doubt) be alcohol-free.

PRO TIP: **LEAVE THE RUM CAKES OUT OF IT!**

While your fellow bakers will enjoy the results of hard work (and a sugar high), this challenge can expand to do good, as well. The proceeds of the bake-off event could be donated to benefit a charity,

Challenge
your friends to put on their thinking caps (and chef hats and aprons, too).

like Alcohol Change UK, or another alcohol-free campaign of your choice. In this way, your temporary abstinence can positively impact other people, in addition to having spillover effects beyond the month on a personal level.

Baby Bottles, Not Spirit Bottles

Baby showers are a time to celebrate a new life stage (and literally another life, or lives, coming soon). Of course, when babies are involved, booze isn't priority No. 1, but if you're planning a shower for a friend, consider that partygoers might want to pop Champagne to commemorate the occasion. Simply replace that bubbly with sparkling cider, and focus on other decorative details. (Guests will respectfully understand it's not the place and time for getting tipsy.)

Even comrades who aren't avoiding alcohol can have a great time without cocktails in hand. Attendees can enjoy themselves without concern for overindulging, embarrassing themselves under the influence, or worrying about getting up early the next morning and trying to be productive.

Food Themes (No, You Can't Bring Fermented Grapes)

The New Year often brings about new diets (but not always). Another creative way to bring friends together is by throwing a food-fest focused on a specific fare. Love potatoes? Cater or make French fries, baked potatoes, potato chips, gnocchi, and more! Apply the same idea to apples and host a shindig with apple pie, apple cobbler, and apple chips! And, as noted earlier, if you (and your friends) are embarking on more restrictive eating, the dishes served at supper can be gluten-free, sugar-free, dairy-free, nut-free, and so on! The choice is yours!

Hot Tea Month

While it's chilly outside, take advantage of frigid temperatures and participate in Hot Tea Month when you're feeling thirsty. While tea time is pretty standard for the Brits, it's not quite as common in the United States and Canada. Get festive with a range of tea flavors—some brands veer from traditional black, Earl Grey, and English Breakfast to fun, creative varieties like cupcake, cookie dough, and cinnamon bun. If you love sweets, don't forget to buy or bake sugary (and savory) scones to pair with your sips. You can prepare small sandwiches, too! Without spirits, beer, and wine, it's a win-win. Speaking of winning, you can also throw a party inspired by real-life winners, actual awards, and heroes . . .

Keeping Score of Drinks: 0–0

Whether cheering on your NFL team during the playoffs or watching your favorite tennis player(s) rally through matches at the Australian Open, there are many, many face-offs to get excited about during winter, especially Dry January–style. Sure, these events are typically viewed with a beverage in hand. But when you throw a no-booze get-together to bond over the game, you and your guests will find it equally refreshing and entertaining without a cold beer or mixed drink. (Which, by the way, totally gets in the way of clapping, shouting, and screaming to encourage the team and discourage the opposing squad—there's definitely an upside to not wearing your favorite beverage by accident.)

For football, hockey, and basketball—no matter your spectator sport—encourage all of your friends to wear the jerseys of players they're cheering for or the colors of the teams they're rooting for. In typical game-day fashion, executing a menu of cheese fries, soda, and wings should keep your guests stuffed, satisfied, and comforted. You can get creative by matching food to the teams' home cities or states. For example, make pizza bagels to represent New York, Chicago dogs for Illinois, and Tex-Mex or barbecue for Texas!

Feeling lucky? Place your bets without being swayed by a few brewskis.

After all, alcohol can instill a sense of overconfidence regarding how things are going (or might turn out). You can better judge your odds from a state of mind that isn't impacted by liquor! Even if you're not a traditional gambler (because you don't want to lose any money, or make your friends pay up), you can place friendly wagers on the game involving bragging rights or who's going to buy your first drink once the month is over!

Golden Globes Gathering

Roll out an actual red carpet for this award show that airs every January! If you're a movie buff, you'll be tuning in to see your favorite stars take home awards (or get snubbed), so why not throw a watch party and invite fellow film fans? For an interactive experience, pass out voting ballots and reward the winner with a gold trophy of his or her own! Get into the theme of the night, and ask your guests to dress up as characters from the movies being honored, or in gowns and tuxedos like the celebs. Instead of taking shots (or a sip of alcohol) each time a certain word or catchphrase is spoken on TV, modify it to fit Dry January by giving guests a gold star sticker each time a sentence starts with "I'd like to thank . . . ," "Who are you wearing?," and the like.

For food, stay on theme with "globes" and purchase or cook sphere-shaped fare. Meatballs, arancini (rice balls), and falafel can serve as passed apps, while cake balls, scooped ice cream, and chocolate truffles are shoo-ins for dessert. Of course, no movie experience is complete without popcorn, so be sure to have that on hand for snacking in between!

PRO TIP: SKIP OUT ON THE "BOOZY" ICE CREAM—OPT FOR ANOTHER DELICIOUS FLAVOR TO KEEP YOUR CHALLENGE COMPLETELY ALCOHOL-FREE.

Model Behavior Monday

Observed on the third Monday in January every year, Martin Luther King Jr. Day is more than an alibi for drinking on that Sunday night— for Dry January participants, the day off from work can be spent in a more productive manner. Organize a get-together in honor of MLK Day! Your party—hosted at a private residence or in a public space— can raise money for charities and organizations supporting equal rights! You can also rally your attendees and "party hop" from community service volunteer opportunities, lectures, and other special events held that day.

No to "Burns Night"

If you're Scottish, of Scottish descent, or if you have an admiration for the Scots (or you happen to be visiting Scotland) on January 25, you may be tempted to participate in Robert Burns Night (or Burns Supper). Inspired by the poet Robert Burns, the evening often involves haggis (a savory Scottish dish—which is actually banned in the United States for utilizing sheeps' lungs), his famed poetry, and lots of Scotch.

BOARD GAMES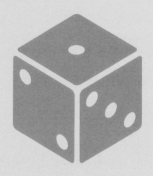

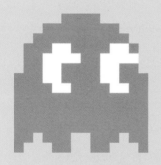 ARCADE GAMES

TV SHOW
CATCHPHRASES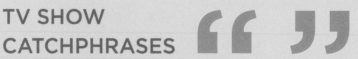

You can choose to participate in these parties without consuming whiskey, or remake your own soiree—sans spirits. In fact, if this date doesn't work for your calendar, create your own poetry night on another evening. You and your guests can recite Burns's works, poems on a chosen theme, and even incorporate personal creative writing pieces into the mix.

Let the Games Be(gin) without Alcohol

Playing board games, participating in card games, going out to compete in arcade games, and attending sports games are great ways to keep yourself (and friends) busy during a dry month. But, if you're still craving another kind of game—dare we say, a drinking game—you can still partake in the fun (with a replacement nonalcoholic liquid). Hear us out: You still won't be boozing, but these contests and matches will keep you from missing out on good-hearted entertainment at home, at bars, or at parties with people who are drinking.

That in itself is a win!

TV SHOW QUOTES OR CATCHPHRASES

In the boozy version of this pastime, participants take a shot or a sip of their drinks every time a character says a specific catchphrase or designated word. The dry format: Instead of taking a shot when characters say certain words or phrases, do a pushup, a crunch, or a pullup (if you have the equipment handy).

PICTURE THIS

In the alcohol-infused mime game, two teams are tasked (one at a time) with creating physical drawings that represent phrases or things. One representative from the team is given a secret word to illustrate. As he or she draws the picture, the teammates must guess what the artwork represents. There is a time limit for each round. With alcohol: If the first team succeeds, the second team drinks, and vice versa. Without booze: The same rules apply—sort of. Replace the standard glass of wine with seltzer, soda, or another N.A. beverage (or make it a betting game with small amounts of cash).

NEVER HAVE I EVER

Well, now things are getting interesting. When drinking is involved in this game, one by one, participants make a statement, admitting "Never have I ever [insert action here]." If any of the other players have done that action at some point in their lives, they take a drink. Rather than throwing back shots or taking a sip of a mixed beverage,

impose a dare that doesn't involve imbibing.

GAMES OF DEXTERITY

With or without a beverage in hand, games like pick-up sticks, Twister, and Jenga require equipment. With an alcoholic beverage at hand, the games progress turn by turn, requiring ever more challenging feats until someone makes a mistake and moves the sticks (pick-up sticks), falls and brings everyone down (Twister), or causes the tower to collapse (Jenga). The person responsible must finish his or her drink. The Dry format: Instead of drinking, the loser is assigned an unwanted chore, pays a small sum of money, or has to tell an embarrassing story about him- or herself.

FLIPCUP

Whether at a sporting event tailgate, a college party, or another outdoor event (read: Things could get sticky . . .), the traditional version (with mixed drinks, spirits, or beer) involves two teams of players who stand across from one another with a table between them. Facing off, each pair of players chug the drink in front of them until it's gone. They place their empty cups on the edge of the table and try to flip them upside down. This action cascades down the line until all players have flipped their containers. You can still play this good ol' classic drinking game—without drinking! Rather than downing booze during the faceoff, try energy drinks, soda, or juice as the beverage component of the match. Oh, and the losing team has to clean up the mess left behind.

WATER PONG

Obviously, the beer-based rendition does not utilize water. Ordinarily known as beer pong, and played with—you guessed it—beer, this standard college party game involves two teams tossing Ping-Pong balls across a long table with the goal of landing the balls inside six to ten cups filled with beer. Once a cup receives a ball, it is removed from the table, and the opposing team must drink the contents inside (beer!). The team who clears all cups first wins. During your N.A. stint, this game is much more hydrating—with H_2O. The losing team has to set up the table for the next game. Raise the stakes by proposing a bet!

Spontaneous No-Reason-Needed Get-Togethers

Maybe an average month doesn't involve baked goods or babies (in the same way it doesn't call for imbibing—both just aren't part of your life at the moment!). Perhaps you're not a movie or sports fan. If sweets or themed get-togethers don't speak to you, that's cool, too! No matter what your schedule or your interests, you don't need an excuse to throw a friendly nonalcoholic brunch, lunch, or dinner party. If you don't have the time to or aren't interested in planning an elaborate shindig, simply throw it together on a whim! Text, call, or email your buddies (hell, send smoke signals if that's your preferred method of communication). Whatever, however, or with as little warning as you want: Do it, and enjoy it!

The point is to see your friends, be social, keep your pact intact, and have as much fun as possible. And, remember: even though you're not drinking, you can still appreciate zero-proof beverages that taste like the real thing. When you're ready to stock your N.A. beverage bar, turn to page 186 for some favorite sip-worthy mocktails.

Bake It 'til You Make It (to the Finish Line)

Substitute attending parties—where alcohol is the main attraction and reason for your attendance—with organizing a themed soiree or get-together of your own, without kegs, liquor handles, and gelatin shots . . . Dry-style!

To help you gather the materials needed for a poppin' party (without popping bottles), brainstorm some ideas using the web (Pinterest is a great starting point for inspiration), and use the handy shopping lists on the right to stay organized!

If you're planning a bake-off, for example (to, you know, replace your liquor calories with delicious, sugary ones!), hosting a shindig full of buttery items may be a bit more comfortable to you than say, lining your friends up for a mocktail competition. (Your squad may have zero experience in both fields, but there's a greater chance they'll know a thing or two about mixing eggs than mixing N.A. drinks . . . maybe.)

There are a variety of goodies to choose from . . . like these delicious recipes from Breads Bakery in New York City to help you roll out delicious treats!

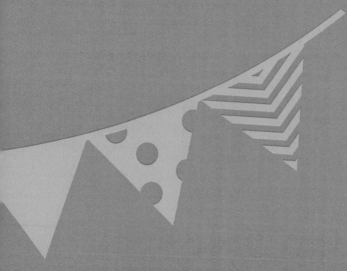

Shopping list for throwing an at-home Bake-Off Bonanza, sans liquor.

BAKED GOODS (see pages 168 to 173 for recipes)
[ ] Challah
[ ] Brownies
[ ] Cookies

DRINKS
[ ] Milk and/or plant-based milks
[ ] Water
[ ] Club soda
[ ] Tea
[ ] Coffee
[ ] Mocktail ingredients
    (see pages 186 to 195 for recipes)

UTENSILS
[ ] Forks
[ ] Knives

DECOR
[ ] Cupcake-themed napkins
[ ] Cake-decorated paper plates
[ ] Balloons with sprinkles

Challah

MAKES 3 LOAVES

Even if you (or your guests) don't have a sweet tooth, you can still indulge in a baked good that won't have them bouncing off the walls: challah! This braided egg bread can be eaten with all meals—even breakfast (where you won't be missing a mimosa)!

PRO TIP: USE IT AS THE BREAD FOR FRENCH TOAST FOR AN EXTRA FLUFFY MORNING TREAT!

FOR THE DOUGH

1 ½ (360 ml) cups water
3 tablespoons fresh yeast
6 (750 g) cups sifted all-purpose flour
2 large eggs
6 tablespoons (75 g) sugar
1 tablespoon salt
¼ cup (60 ml) sunflower seed oil, corn oil, or melted butter

FOR THE GLAZE

1 egg, beaten
Sesame and poppy seeds

1. Make the dough: Pour the water into the bowl of a stand mixer and crumble the yeast into the water. Add the flour, eggs, sugar, salt, and oil in that order.

2. Attach the dough hook and mix on low speed for 4 minutes to combine. Increase the speed to medium and knead for another 5 minutes, or until a soft, smooth dough is formed.

3. Remove the dough to a lightly floured work surface, and roll into a ball. Place the ball of dough in a lightly floured bowl. Cover the bowl with a kitchen towel or plastic wrap and let rise at room temperature until almost doubled in volume, about 40 minutes.

4. Line a baking sheet with parchment paper. Using a knife, divide the dough into 3 equal portions and then divide each portion into three pieces (a total of 9). For each loaf, roll 3 pieces of dough into logs 10 inches (25 cm) long. Connect the 3 logs at one end and braid to the other end. Transfer the loaf to the lined baking sheet. Repeat to make 3 loaves.

5. Cover the loaves with a kitchen towel and let rise at room temperature until doubled, about 35 minutes.

6. Meanwhile, preheat the oven to 425°F.

7. Glaze the loaves: Once the challahs have doubled in volume, gently brush them with the beaten egg and generously sprinkle with sesame and poppy seeds.

8. Bake until golden brown, about 25 minutes.

9. Remove from the oven and cool.

Flourless Brownie Cake

MAKES 3 BROWNIE CAKES

Whether you're "treating yourself" after a long week or observing a momentous occasion, neither require the involvement of booze in a glass, from a bottle, or included in a dessert on a plate. Ditch the rum cake and rum raisin ice cream for a sweet that will keep you alcohol-free and feeling celebratory.

1 ⅔ cups (290 g) dark chocolate chips (70% cacao)
1 ½ sticks (6 ounces) + 1 tablespoon (185 g) unsalted butter
4 large eggs
1 cup + 1 tablespoon (215 g) granulated sugar
¼ cup + 1 tablespoon (140 g) cornstarch
¼ cup + 1 tablespoons (175 g) potato starch
1 teaspoon baking powder

1. Position a rack in the center of the oven and preheat the oven to 350°F (175°C). Spray the edges of a 9x3x1-inch (23x7.5x2.5 cm) aluminum tray with cooking spray and line the bottom with parchment paper.

2. In a double boiler or a heatproof bowl set over a pot of simmering water, melt the chocolate.

3. In a small saucepan, bring the butter to a low boil. Once the butter boils, immediately remove from the heat and add the butter to the melted chocolate. Using a whisk, constantly mix by hand for 3 minutes. Set aside.

4. In a stand mixer fitted with the whisk, combine the eggs and sugar and mix for 2 minutes. Once the eggs and sugar are combined, slowly pour in the chocolate mixture and mix on low speed for 3 minutes.

5. In a separate bowl, sift together the cornstarch, potato starch, and baking powder. With the mixer on low speed, add the dry ingredients and mix for 1 minute. Using a rubber spatula, scrape down the bowl and continue to mix on low speed for 2 more minutes, ensuring all the dry ingredients are completely mixed in and there are no lumps.

6 Pour the batter into the lined pan and, using an offset spatula, spread the batter evenly in the whole pan.

7. Transfer to the oven and immediately lower the oven temperature to 325°F (165°C). Bake until the cake is firm but has a slight jiggle, 15 to 18 minutes. It should no longer look wet and shiny on top.

8. Allow the brownie cake to cool completely before cutting and serving.

Chocolate Chip Cookies

MAKES 36 COOKIES

Here's a throwback to a childhood favorite! Rather than pairing a meal with a fine glass of wine for these chocolate chip cookies, all you need is any type of milk to accompany this sweet snack! Whether it's traditional milk, soy, oat, or almond (or any other type), dip a chocolate chip cookie in your cold beverage for a trip down memory lane.

PRO TIP: IF YOU'D LIKE TO SAVE SOME DOUGH FOR A LATER TIME, YOU CAN FREEZE THE DOUGH FOR UP TO 3 MONTHS. WHEN READY TO BAKE, ALLOW THE DOUGH TO COMPLETELY THAW BEFORE BAKING.

2 cups (340 g) dark chocolate discs
2 cups (340 g) milk chocolate discs
½ cup (85 g) white chocolate discs
1 tablespoon all-purpose flour
2 sticks (8 ounces) + 2 tablespoons (255 g) unsalted butter
⅔ (135 g) cup granulated sugar
1 cup + ⅓ cup (195 g) packed dark brown sugar
3 large eggs
4 cups pastry flour
2 teaspoons baking powder
1¼ teaspoons salt

1. Preheat the oven to 300°F (150°C). Line a large baking sheet with parchment paper.

2. In a food processor, combine the chocolates with the 1 tablespoon all-purpose flour. Pulse until coarsely chopped. Set aside.

3. In a stand mixer fitted with the paddle attachment, combine the butter, granulated sugar, and brown sugar. Beat on high speed for 10 minutes. Using a rubber spatula, scrape down the sides of the bowl and the paddle. Continue to mix on high speed for 1 minute.

4. On low speed, add the eggs one at a time, allowing each egg to be completely mixed in before adding the next. Once all the eggs are completely mixed in, scrape down the bowl and paddle and mix on low speed for 1 minute.

5. In a separate bowl, sift together the pastry flour, baking powder, and salt. Add ⅓ of the dry ingredients at a time to the mixer and mix on low speed until completely incorporated before adding the next portion. Scrape the bowl and paddle and mix on low speed for an additional 30 seconds to 1 minute, ensuring all the dry ingredients have been mixed in properly.

6. On low speed, gradually beat in the chopped chocolate and mix for 30 seconds. Turn off the mixer and hand-mix the dough, ensuring all the ingredients are completely mixed.

7. Scoop ⅓ cup of cookie dough onto the lined baking sheet. Bake until cookies are golden brown all over and look slightly puffed up in the center, 15 to 18 minutes, rotating the pan front to back halfway through.

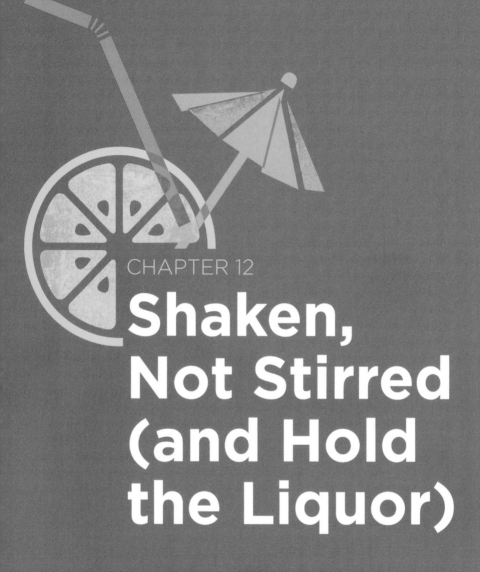

CHAPTER 12

Shaken, Not Stirred (and Hold the Liquor)

If you love the taste of a great, well-balanced cocktail or an ice-cold beer, but you aren't drinking alcohol (perhaps you're mid-month, and you're still exercising your right to abstain), you can still enjoy a mixed, muddled, shaken, stirred, or bottled nonalcoholic beverage. (Hallelujah!)

Get creative by making mocktails, requesting N.A. beverages at bars and restaurants, or buying faux beers and elixirs in stores and online.

Make Your Own

Mocktails (aka nonalcoholic mixed drinks) are beverages that taste like cocktails but don't involve beer, wine, or spirits—at all. Many N.A. concoctions call for all the same ingredients (minus the booze, of course) that you'd find on a cocktail menu: fruit, juice, purees, ice, syrups (simple and other), and tonic—and more can be incorporated, according to your taste. Before you take your first sip, top off your creation with a fun, tasty, and photogenic garnish (or multiple garnishes). Get artsy with cinnamon sticks, candied ginger, apple slices, orange peels, or even pickles (depending on the cocktail—perhaps save the latter for a nonhangover-inducing booze-free Bloody Mary).

While sipping, you definitely won't feel tipsy, but you might want to take a picture or two . . . hell, go crazy and make an entire photo album. Upload those pics to social media if you'd like. And, as a reminder to all of your Sober Month Support Squad buddies (and people you've made friendly, or real, bets with), don't forget to add #dryjanuary in the caption (if it is, in fact, January . . . and not another dry month) as a token of loyalty to your commitment. These N.A. beverages are going to look so good that you might fool a few followers into thinking you gave into the temptation of tequila!

There are a bunch of N.A. beverage recipe books that instruct how to make, prepare, and serve mocktails. Even more popular are food, beverage, and lifestyle websites with articles that feature delicious, refreshing, and satisfying zero-proof cocktails and punches. Tap into your favorite search engine to get lost in an overwhelming list of options (in a good way)! Or, you can turn to page 186 for tasty sips.

Unless you prefer to eyeball it (read: make an educated guess), your booze-free-beverage best friend is going to be a jigger. A jigger is a simple measuring tool usually used for assigning quantities of liquor (but also employed to gauge amounts of other ingredients, too). This will be especially helpful to you for measuring accuracy (and therefore, balance and tastiness).

Other helpful utensils are:

Cocktail shaker A shaker is a vessel that helps you mix your beverages (as the name suggests) by shaking them together. There are two parts to it: a metal cup (see mixing tin, below) and either a lid or another cup that works as a lid.

Mixing tin This is a large metal cup, usually part of a shaker, but it can be used alone, too.

Strainer When the contents of a drink are shaken in a shaker with ice, the drink is poured into a cup or glass through a strainer, which separates the ice from the mixed drink by holding it back in the shaker.

Muddler A muddler helps you mash up ingredients like fruit, smushing them between the muddler's end piece and your glass.

Bar spoon A bar spoon has a long handle, and the actual spoon part holds the volume of a teaspoon.

Ice bucket An ice bucket holds your ice.

There are more tools that can help you achieve delicious drinks, but these are the basics.

Your
booze-free-beverage
best friend
is going to be a

jigger

After you've tested a few tried-and-true mocktails, go rogue and make your own! As with cooking and baking, you can modify an existing classic or be your own favorite N.A. bartender and invent a new formula!

STILL, SPARKLING, OR DISTILLED (BUT STILL NOT ALCOHOL)

Another piece to Dry January's mocktail recipe puzzle is the inclusion of nonalcoholic bottled components. You can buy premade virgin Bloody Mary, daiquiri, and other mixes at the store or on the Internet—and never add the booze to your cart or your beverage. Instead, add H_2O, sparkling water, or another carbonated liquid (such as a lemon-lime soda for margaritas).

- Fever-Tree and Q Drinks produce mixers for traditional cocktails, but these can both be used as supplements for N.A. beverages (after all, they contain zero alcohol).
- Although spirits are the base (read: the shining stars!) in traditional cocktails, N.A. mixed drinks replace bourbon, gin, mezcal, and more with booze-free elements and brands such as Curious Elixirs or Seedlip—as well as teas or just still, sparkling, or distilled water.

Curious Elixirs combine herbs, barks, spices, botanicals, and roots with organic juices. The result is a lightly carbonated, flavorful 11.2-ounce drink without added sugar, gluten, dairy, and nuts (or alcohol!). You can order a variety of flavors, and search the web for recipes to keep you sipping through the month.

Seedlip is a distilled nonalcoholic spirit specially made to be served mixed with tonic or within mocktails. Not only is it zero proof, but Seedlip is also calorie- and sugar-free. Even though it's bottled and blended in England, Seedlip is not exclusive to the UK. It's available to nonimbibing patrons both online and in person at notable bars in the United States, including True Laurel and Che Fico in San Francisco; Michelin-star restaurants Eleven Madison Park and The NoMad in New York City; and BLVD, Cindy's, and The Aviary in Chicago.

Kin Euphorics, another nonalcoholic beverage, launched in 2018. Promising to elevate your state, it contains adaptogens, nootropics, and botanics (rather than boozy components). High Rhode (aka Hibiscus Rhodiola) has notes of earthy florals, tart citrus, and warming spice with a bite. Poured over ice or topped with soda, it can be enjoyed by anyone over eighteen (who isn't pregnant, trying to get pregnant, or breastfeeding).

- Large corporations are looking for a piece of N.A. beverage sales, too. In January 2019 (yes, right in time for thirty-one drink-free days), Coca-Cola rolled out BAR NØNE, a line of nonalcoholic cocktail-inspired beverages in its hometown of Atlanta, to test its popularity. Coca-Cola isn't the only business getting into alcohol-inspired sips: Beer brands are, too (more on that later, on page 182).
- Beverages containing cannabidiol, more commonly known as CBD, are becoming increasingly popular in drink form. CBD is used to treat anxiety and insomnia. Some brands infuse CBD into sparkling water, tea, or coffee. It is also sold separately as a liquid and can be manually added (with an eyedropper) to any N.A. beverage of choice.

Hit the Bar (but Not the Booze)

While Dry January has been a part of pop culture in the UK for years, the concept is a little newer in the United States. But rest assured, participants in the States can feel comfortable going to bars, specifically without dreading alienating drink menus that don't cater to N.A. needs. Instead, bartenders and beverage directors (you know, the people who plan the drink menus) in such cities as New York, Chicago, Los Angeles, and San Francisco have adapted to the Dry January movement by offering creative and re-created classic concoctions without an alcoholic component.

In addition, a variety of destinations known for imbibing have also stocked their refrigerators with nonalcoholic beer and wine alternatives. So even if mixed drinks aren't your thing, there's something for everyone to enjoy!

DRY STATE(S) OF MIND

When places that serve booze have mocktails available, it encourages the consumer to abstain from boozy bevs while socializing, and the venue still earns cash for the bar that might otherwise miss out on a sale.

For example, even Las Vegas—an over-the-top city attracting hard-partying tourists—has adapted to its nonimbibing visitors. At The Dorsey, a chic cocktail lounge located on the casino floor of the Venetian Hotel, N.A. beverages are menu staples. "Nonalcoholic menu options make bars more inclusive to all guests and their preferences," says Juyoung Kang, lead bartender at The Dorsey (check page 187 for her recipe). Kang says they're not just making fruit punch cocktails with cranberry, orange, and pineapple juices. She adds,

"We're using our creativity and a bit of science, at times, to make something ordinary, extraordinary."

Meanwhile, Otium, a contemporary restaurant in downtown Los Angeles, caters to the needs of Dry January participants each year. Three drinks on its cocktail menu can be converted to N.A. offerings using a distilled nonalcoholic spirit, while two other drinks are specifically crafted and offered without booze. Patrons can also order a "bartender's choice" N.A. beverage, made with ingredients the venue has on hand.

"It's important for us that we treat our guests who don't drink alcohol with the same respect as imbibers," says Chris Amirault, bar program director at Otium. "There should be an equal amount of effort and creativity that goes into cocktails without booze as those with it."

Amirault recognizes the thirty-one dry days of January have become a huge trend in the industry and the Greater Los Angeles area as a whole.

"Guests who don't imbibe are more likely to order N.A. beverages if they feel like the bartenders care about their needs as well," says Amirault, who acknowledges that Dry Jan increases the volume of N.A. beverage orders "pretty considerably" during the chilly month. "Taking care of your body is something most Angelenos care greatly about. Dry Jan is a perfect time for people to take an inventory with themselves to reset and refocus, and I think eliminating alcohol is a great way to start."

50 PERCENT MOCKTAILS AND 50 PERCENT COCKTAILS, 100 PERCENT OF THE TIME

At some traditional alcohol-serving establishments, mocktails are a key element that draws customers in. Vena's Fizz House, in Portland, Maine, is a cocktail/mocktail bar and mixology shop that gives N.A. and boozy beverages equal real estate on the menu. Nonalcoholic beverages for purchase include Fizzes, Old Fashioned Sippers, Lemonades, Lime Rickeys, Seedlip Mocktails, Herbal Spritzers, Botanical Mocktails, and more.

BOOZE-FREE BARS

Venues dedicated to zero-proof drinks have popped up, too. At Getaway Bar in Brooklyn, mixed drinks incorporate alcohol-free spirits (like Seedlip), drinking vinegars, and less-commonly recognized sodas to create unique flavor combinations. Of course, everything on site has 0 ABV. Booze-free Listen Bar started as a one-time pop-up. It evolved into a bar that is open one night each month in Manhattan's East Village. The entire menu was crafted without alcohol, wine, or beer (although nonalcoholic spirits are used in mixed drinks, and nonalcoholic beer is served)! And in East Brooklyn's Bushwick neighborhood, Ambrosia Elixirs is a botanical cafe and apothecary bar known for hand-crafted botanical elixirs, herbal tinctures, and tonics.

KAVA, NOT CAVA

Not to be mistaken with Cava, Spanish sparkling wine, kava (obviously with a "K") is a nonalcoholic beverage that (upon consumption) is known for its sedative properties, namely lessening anxiety and promoting relaxation. Kava Lounge in San Francisco and SquareRut Kava Bar in Austin, Texas, serve the herbal remedy in liquid form, as beverages.

Buying Nonboozy Beverages and Sober-Friendly Supplements

Sure, opting for water is a great way to stay hydrated. Sipping fruit juice can satisfy a sweet tooth and help you consume important vitamins. Even ordering a soda will keep your hands occupied during happy hours. But in addition to drinking those regular, everyday liquids, there are beers, ciders, wines (and more) that taste just like your favorite boozy beverages (without alcohol) and won't hijack your dry month.

BEERS WITHOUT A BUZZ

For beer fans: Peroni, Heineken, Guinness, Coors, and Budweiser have their own lesser-known N.A. versions, while Anheuser-Busch's O'Doul's might sound familiar.

(PS: you can drink as much as you'd like without repercussions such as a nasty hangover or tipsy texting!)

For reference: de-alcoholized beer contains no more than 0.5 percent ABV. And, although marketed as nonalcoholic beers, "alcohol-free" beer technically could contain trace amounts of alcohol (less than 0.05 percent). So if you're 100 percent committed to a totally sober month, read your labels wisely! These advertising tactics aren't trying to trick you. The reality is, some alcohol is naturally created during the brewing process, but it's very, very minimal.

"Nonalcoholic beer is made basically the same way alcoholic beer is made: with water, malt, hops, yeast, brewing process, yadda-yadda," says Adam Vavrick, the beer director for the Publican, Publican Tavern, and Publican Quality Meats in Chicago. "Fermentation creates alcohol, so we gotta get it out of there!"

He says there are three main methods of removing alcohol from beer—**heat, reverse osmosis, and vacuum distillation**—used either alone or in some combination. Each has a drawback, but all are tried-and-true ways to create an N.A. brewski.

Heat: Alcohol boils at a lower temperature than water, so you can drive it off by heating the beer above 173.5°F, causing the alcohol to evaporate. This is the old-school method. You can also technically do this at home if you're a home brewer: Make the beer as you normally do (but with way fewer hops), ferment it, and then, when the process is completed, put the beer back in your kettle. Heat it to 174°F-ish for 30 minutes, then chill it back down and keg as you normally would. There is no bottling option here (unless you're a brewery), because if you add priming sugar and yeast, you're just going to create more alcohol. *The drawback to the heat method is that it drives off all those wonderful flavors and aromas of beer, much to the detriment of the finished product.*

Reverse osmosis: This is where you pass the finished beer through some sort of semipermeable membrane, usually under pressure. Think of it like pushing liquid through a filter with very, very small holes. These holes are so small they (almost) only allow water and alcohol to pass through. All of the proteins, hop oils, and so on don't make it through and stay as part of the "retentate" (a fancy name for beer sludge). The water and alcohol that passed through the filter (now called "permeate") has its alcohol removed by the heat method (that you just read about) or vacuum distillation (which you're going to learn about in one minute), and this is then added back to the retentate, with or without additional water, to make the finished alcohol-free beer. You're basically separating the "beer" from the "not beer" parts, adjusting one element, and then mixing them back up. *The downside? Using extra equipment is expensive and it's a finicky process.*

Vacuum distillation: The process uses the same principle as the heat method, but conducted in a vacuum, which drastically lowers the temperature required to get the ethanol (a simple alcohol) to be driven off. The stronger the vacuum, the lower the boiling point. The theory here is that a lower boiling point keeps more of those volatiles (like hop oils and such) in the finished product. This method is usually used in conjunction with reverse osmosis for a gentler approach to boiling. *The not-so-good news: It takes a lot of expensive equipment and a vacuum powerful enough to make an appreciable difference in temperature, and no doubt the energy costs go up, too!*

Vavrick notes that legally in the United States, nonalcoholic beer can have up to 0.5 percent ABV. Most labels list this percentage. Barring a lab test, it's best to consult the brewery!

And that's your science lecture on how N.A. beer is made!

CIDER (SANS SLURRING)

Hard ciders, begone! (At least during designated dry weeks!) Both alcoholic and nonalcoholic ciders are produced by crushing fruit. Most of the time, they're made from apples—but not always. Chain grocers like Trader Joe's and Safeway sell their own brands of N.A. sparkling ciders, and staple brands like Martinelli's offer a range of flavors including apple-cranberry, apple-pear, apple-peach, and more. If you have a craving, these N.A. ciders are great alternatives to the boozy kind and also an easy swap for sparkling wine!

IT'S TIME FOR (N.A.) WINE!

Aka Wine:30. Puns aside, just as there are nonalcoholic cocktails, beers, and ciders, there are a variety of wine brands that you can cheers with during your thirty-one-day challenge. ARIEL produces dealcoholized wines, including Chardonnay and Cabernet Sauvignon, made from grapes grown in California. Some of the brand's dealcoholized varietals are aged in small oak barrels before being fined (which removes unwanted material) and filtered. After these traditional winemaking methods, the wine is then put through a cold filtration process (which uses reverse osmosis, for you science-y people!), in which more than 99.5 percent of the alcohol is removed.

N.A. Chardonnay drinkers can also opt for St. Regis Chardonnay, a medium-bodied wine with floral and fruity aromas (and less than 0.5 percent alcohol).

Sparkling wine aficionados can rejoice over flutes filled with Fre Brut Alcohol-Removed Sparkling Wine from Sutter Home. And rosé fanatics can sip Pierre Zéro Nonalcoholic Rosé from Pierre Chavin or their Pierre Sparkling Rosé—both contain zero-percent alcohol.

When real wine, beer, and cocktails aren't an option during Dry January, or any other booze-free period, there are many options for similar-tasting possibilities to experiment with. Sipping, chugging, and even taking shots won't get anyone drunk (or even buzzed)! You may develop a sugar high (depending on the contents of your drink), but you can still stay sober for the month. **Cheers to that!**

Hooray for N.A. Beverage Recipes!

One month of sobriety means no cocktails . . . but mocktails? Those are totally kosher by dry-month standards. Create these nonalcoholic, tasty, thirst-quenching mixed drinks at home. Or, if you're out-and-about in the cities where they've been featured on menus, pop by these bars and restaurants and order a round (or two, or three).

Stone Fruit Season

Even if you're headed to the city of sin, you don't have to drink. Evan Hosaka, lead bartender at Electra Cocktail Club in Las Vegas, created a Tiki-style cocktail that you'll enjoy if you're into Mai Tais, Zombies, or Singapore Slings.

SERVES 1
GLASS: COLLINS

2 ounces (60 ml) pineapple juice
1 ounce (30 ml) peach puree
¾ ounce (23 ml) fresh lime juice
¾ ounce (23 ml) honey syrup
   (5 parts honey:1 part water)
1 dropper of Hellfire habanero shrub

Crushed ice
Dash of club soda (optional)
1 parasol, for garnish

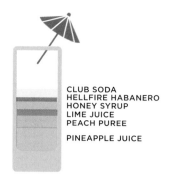

CLUB SODA
HELLFIRE HABANERO
HONEY SYRUP
LIME JUICE
PEACH PUREE

PINEAPPLE JUICE

In a cocktail shaker, combine the pineapple juice, peach puree, lime juice, honey syrup, and shrub. Shake vigorously. Fill the glass with ice. Strain the drink into the glass. Top with club soda if desired. Garnish with a parasol.

Garden Party

If you're craving a Mojito or a daiquiri, Juyoung Kang, lead bartender at The Dorsey in Las Vegas, has a recipe for a bright and refreshing N.A. beverage. Even in the cooler months, this mocktail will transport you to sunnier days.

SERVES 1
GLASS: COLLINS

Ice
2 ounces (60 ml) fresh green apple juice
1 ounce (30 ml) fresh cucumber juice
½ ounce (15 ml) fresh lime juice
½ ounce (15 ml) simple syrup
10 mint leaves
2 ounces (60 ml) club soda
Ice
3 to 4 half-moon slices green apples, for garnish

In an ice-filled cocktail shaker, combine the apple juice, cucumber juice, lime juice, simple syrup, and mint leaves. Shake vigorously. Add the club soda to the shaker and strain into an ice-filled glass. Garnish with the green apples.

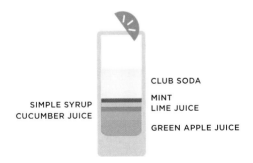

SIMPLE SYRUP
CUCUMBER JUICE

CLUB SODA

MINT
LIME JUICE

GREEN APPLE JUICE

Summer Sling

Admittedly, you can complete sober months outside of January (and October, too). If you choose to challenge yourself in the summer months, this N.A. drink by Nicholas Krok, director of nightlife at 1 Hotel Brooklyn Bridge, will keep you satisfied in warm weather. It tastes like a tiki bar cocktail made friends with a watermelon. (You know, gotta love new friends.)

SERVES 1
GLASS: COLLINS

4 slices cucumber
1 ½ ounces (45 ml) simple syrup (made with evaporated cane juice)
1 ½ ounces (45 ml) fresh lemon juice
1 ounce (30 ml) organic pineapple juice
4 dashes of peach bitters
Crushed ice
2 ounces (60 ml) club soda
1 teaspoon grenadine
1 lime wheel and 1 cherry, for garnish

In a cocktail shaker, muddle the cucumber with the simple syrup. Add the lemon juice, pineapple juice, and bitters. Shake hard for about 8 seconds. Fill the glass with crushed ice and add the soda. Strain the drink into the glass and garnish with the grenadine, a lime wheel, and cherry.

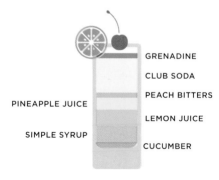

GRENADINE

CLUB SODA

PEACH BITTERS

PINEAPPLE JUICE

LEMON JUICE

SIMPLE SYRUP

CUCUMBER

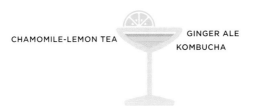

CHAMOMILE-LEMON TEA

GINGER ALE
KOMBUCHA

French 76 on the Detox Tip

With refreshing and detoxing elements, this beverage leaves you with a ginger surprise. It is a mocktail version of the vodka and Champagne French 75 classic and was created by Adrian Mishek, director of restaurant operations at W Washington, DC. If you like margaritas, you will like this because it's bright and colorful, full of flavor, and has a hint of spice.

SERVES 1
GLASS: LEOPOLD COUPE

3 ounces (90 ml) Blue Ridge Bucha Elderflower Sunrise kombucha
2 ounces (60 ml) chilled chamomile-lemon tea
1 ounce (30 ml) Fever-Tree ginger ale
1 lemon peel

1. Pour the kombucha and tea into cocktail mixing glass. Stir until cold.

2. Pour chilled mixture into Leopold coupe.

3. Top off with the ginger ale and garnish with the lemon peel

Spiced Maple Mule

If Moscow Mules are your thing, try this nonalcoholic version with a twist. Nicholas Krok, director of nightlife at 1 Hotel Brooklyn Bridge, concocted an N.A. recipe that tastes as though the classic Mule learned how to bake.

SERVES 1
GLASS: COPPER MUG

4 ounces (120 ml) Spiced Maple Syrup (recipe follows)
4 ounces (120 ml) fresh lime juice
Ginger beer
Ice
Cinnamon stick, for garnish

In a copper mug, combine the syrup and lime juice and give a quick stir. Add ginger beer to taste and ice to fill the mug. Garnish with a cinnamon stick.

Spiced Maple Syrup

MAKES 1½ CUPS (360 ML)

1 cup (240 ml) pure maple syrup
½ cup (120 ml) filtered water
1 star anise
6 whole cloves
4 allspice berries
1 cinnamon stick
10 black peppercorns

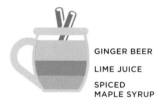

GINGER BEER

LIME JUICE

SPICED
MAPLE SYRUP

In a saucepan, combine the maple syrup, water, star anise, cloves, allspice, cinnamon stick, and black peppercorns and bring to a boil over high heat, stirring regularly. Remove from the heat and let steep for 15 minutes or until desired spice flavor is reached. Let cool. Strain out the spices.

Grove & Garden Tonic

For a Paloma-like zero-proof drink, Nicholas Krok, director of Nightlife at 1 Hotel Brooklyn Bridge, has a recipe that is reminiscent of a fresh spring day. Because, you know, after winter (and months after Dry January) comes spring! So, here's a mocktail to keep you reaching for booze if you decide to prolong your sober days into the next season.

SERVES 1
GLASS: COLLINS

1 ounce (30 ml) fresh lime juice plus more for the glass
salt
⅛ red bell pepper
1½ ounces (45 ml) Black Pepper Agave Syrup (recipe follows)
1 ounce (30 ml) fresh grapefruit juice
2 to 3 ounces (60–90 ml) tonic water
Ice
Thin grapefruit wedges, for garnish

1. Line the glass by dipping the rim in lime juice, followed by salt.

2. In a cocktail shaker, muddle the bell pepper with the agave syrup. Add 1 ounce (30 ml) lime juice and the grapefruit juice and shake hard for 8 seconds. Fill the glass with ice and add the tonic. Top with the shaken ingredients.

3. Garnish with a grapefruit wedge.

Black Pepper Agave Syrup

MAKES 1½ CUPS (360 ML)

1 cup (240 ml) blue Weber agave syrup
½ cup (120 ml) filtered water
20 to 30 black peppercorns

TONIC

GRAPEFRUIT
JUICE
RED PEPPER
LIME JUICE

BLACK
PEPPER
AGAVE
SYRUP

In a saucepan, combine the agave syrup, water, and peppercorns and bring to a boil over high heat, stirring regularly. Immediately remove from the heat and let steep for about 15 minutes or until the desired pepper flavor is reached. Strain out peppercorns.

Weeping Willow

At the W Atlanta Midtown, bartender Debbie Jo makes a mocktail for people who prefer Palomas. The colorful drink offers a refreshing taste, minus the booze! (P.S., No tears here, like the name suggests!)

SERVES 1
GLASS: WHITE WINE GLASS

3 raspberries
3 blackberries
Ice
2 ounces (60 ml) grapefruit juice
2 ½ ounces (75 ml) peach puree
1 ounce (30 ml) simple syrup
Tonic water
Mint leaves

1. In a cocktail shaker, muddle the raspberries and blackberries. Add ice to the shaker. Add the grapefruit juice, peach puree, and simple syrup and shake vigorously.

2. Strain into an ice-filled white wine glass. Top with tonic water. Garnish with mint leaves.

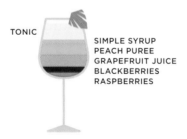

TONIC

SIMPLE SYRUP
PEACH PUREE
GRAPEFRUIT JUICE
BLACKBERRIES
RASPBERRIES

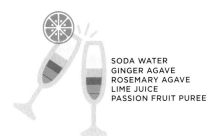

SODA WATER
GINGER AGAVE
ROSEMARY AGAVE
LIME JUICE
PASSION FRUIT PUREE

Nectar of the Gods

*If you like fruity cocktails, Amanda Thomas, bar chef at SoBou,
W New Orleans - French Quarter has a mocktail just for you. The
easy-to-create N.A. beverage will satisfy your desire for a sweet sip.*

SERVES 1
GLASS: CHAMPAGNE FLUTE

Ice
½ ounce (15 ml) passion fruit puree
½ ounce (15 ml) fresh lime juice
½ ounce (15 ml) rosemary agave
½ ounce (15 ml) ginger agave
Soda water
1 orange peel, for garnish

In an ice-filled cocktail shaker, combine the passion fruit puree, lime
juice, and both agaves. Shake vigorously. Strain into a Champagne
flute. Top with soda water. Garnish with the orange peel.

SPICY AF

As the name suggests, this mocktail resembles a spicy margarita (unspiked, of course). The Vita Coco creation is best for an N.A. fiesta and paired with a bold attitude.

SERVES 1
GLASS: LOWBALL

Ice
½ lime
12 ounces Super Sparkling by Vita Coco, Lemon Ginger
1 dash habanero bitters
Jalapeno slices, for garnish

Fill the glass with ice. Squeeze two lime wedges over the ice. Add Super Sparkling by Vita Coco, Lemon Ginger to the glass. Add a dash of habanero bitters. Garnish with jalapeno slices.

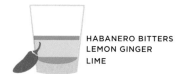

HABANERO BITTERS
LEMON GINGER
LIME

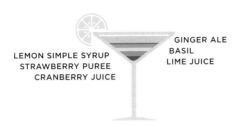

LEMON SIMPLE SYRUP
STRAWBERRY PUREE
CRANBERRY JUICE

GINGER ALE
BASIL
LIME JUICE

Garnet Gimlet

Even if you're "so over" holiday-colored cocktails, you can still celebrate after "the most wonderful time of the year" with a colorful mocktail. For those who enjoy gimlets, sours, or daiquiris, Megan Ardizoni, beverage director at Beauty & Essex in New York City, dreamed up a drink that will have you uploading pics to social media to show off your skills.

SERVES 1
GLASS: MARTINI

Ice
2 ounces (60 ml) white cranberry juice
1 ½ ounces (45 ml) strawberry puree
¾ ounce (23 ml) lemon simple syrup
1 ounce (30 ml) fresh lime juice
3 large basil leaves, shredded
Ginger ale
1 lemon wedge, for garnish

In an ice-filled cocktail shaker, combine the cranberry juice, strawberry puree, lemon simple syrup, lime juice, and basil leaves. Shake vigorously. Strain into a martini glass. Add a splash of ginger ale. Garnish with a lemon wedge.

CHAPTER 13

In Case of Hiccups, Break Glass (Figuratively)

Okay, okay—admittedly—as a human being, you're not perfect. Totally understand (truthfully, no one is!). People make mistakes and slip up from time to time. In most instances, mess-ups can be forgiven and (if you're lucky) even remedied. A dry month is not an exception to this rule.

Your month-long no-drinking stint doesn't have to end completely if you have a rough start easing into it, if you happen to yield to peer pressure midway through, or even if you mess up toward the end. With any major lifestyle change, like completely cutting out alcohol, there's a bit of a transition—or at least, a learning curve.

Caution: Slippery When Wet (Options for How to Get Back Up)

While breaking your pledge isn't ideal—it's life! These things happen. Have no fear: It's certainly forgivable (unlike forgetting your best friend's birthday, which, by the way: totally not cool). Please know you can continue to participate in your month-long challenge, regardless of any slip-ups, if you're willing to revisit the no-booze party bus. There are ways to push onward with the challenge, and opportunities for drink-free do-overs throughout the year. While momentarily breaking (more accurately: pausing) your dry month isn't ideal, adapt! (And good for you for bouncing back, and not calling it quits altogether.) You're already on the path to success!

ONE-DRINK AND ONE-SIP SITUATIONS

For the sake of feeling less constrained (or feeling less guilty), some people who partake in dry months opt for a one-drink option. For example, during "One-Drink January," participants allow themselves to splurge on one drink (as the name suggests) for the entirety of the thirty-one days. This amendment lightens the pressure a bit (even if Dry Jan participants never cash in on the exception). And even if you stumble a little (maybe more than one drink or more than one night out on the town), you don't have to give up your efforts completely! This month isn't about punishing yourself; it's about accomplishing your personal goal(s). Your one-drink-free pass can also be considered authorization for multiple drinks within one twenty-four-hour period (aka One–Drinking-Day January, if you fancy). The same rule of leniency applies to Sober October (One-Sip October), or any other otherwise alcohol-free month.

Most omit (or don't even acknowledge, or know about) this one-beverage option, but it could come in handy for a special occasion that isn't going to happen ever again (like, ever again). The no-lager loophole can be redeemed for a friend's birthday, a wedding, a celebration (like a new job or a promotion), a special reunion (with family or friends), or any random night of the week (here's looking at you, Friday!).

So if you are participating in a dry month where you're abstaining from alcohol, *and* getting married during that time period—congrats! No one expects (or demands) you to be completely alcohol-free at your own wedding. This is a time to raise a glass (or two, or three) to starting a new chapter with your soulmate! Cheers to that. It's a celebration, and you don't have to restrict yourself or feel guilty about drinking during this once-in-a-lifetime event. If you want to drink, do it! If you don't want to drink, go right ahead and skip it. If you want to limit yourself to a certain number of Champagnes or restrict your visits to the open bar, that's cool, too. This day is your day (and of course your spouse's, too), and you should carry on with the day or night as you wish. (And again—yay! Congrats! So happy for you!)

In the same vein, if you're a bridesmaid or a groomsman, and your sister, brother, BFF, college roommate—whatever, whoever—is getting married, celebrate with them, dammit! Drink what you want, or don't drink at all (remember: Soda water can be your perfect plus-one), but don't let your dry-month limitations or rules get in the way of a fun time. You can definitely continue on the same path the very next day!

PAUSE

PRO TIP: **PACE YOURSELF! ESPECIALLY IF YOU'RE NEARING THE END OF A DRY MONTH, YOUR ALCOHOL TOLERANCE WON'T BE AS STRONG AS IT WAS IN DECEMBER. FOR MORE SAFETY—AND HANGOVER—TIPS, CHECK OUT PAGE 209.**

But once the one-drink day, night, or singular beverage is finished (even if you don't empty your beer can), it's back to business as usual—no wine, beer, or spirits until the month is over. And, if you're feeling like you want that one day back on your side, simply extend your challenge to February 2 to make up for lost time!

It's also important to note that your one drink in January doesn't have to be planned in advance. If you're in the moment, and having a good time with friends, enjoy yourself then and there. Sometimes spontaneous drinks happen without the slightest notice or any advance warning (like, engagements or a breakup). Of course, we urge you to resist, but if that's not in the cards, that's okay. Don't shame yourself for succumbing—simply resolve that you'll do better tomorrow and every day moving forward.

FALSE START? MAKE THE MOST OF THE NEXT MONTH

If January just wasn't working out for you (for whatever reason), give February a shot (a chance, that is). Giving up alcohol during month No. 2 won't be Dry January (for obvious reasons), but it does still count as a month without booze. And unlike January, February has only twenty-eight (sometimes twenty-nine) days, making your challenge two to three days shorter. The same goes for any other month.

If Sober October doesn't pan out for you as planned, fret not. Restart your challenge and gear up for a November with no alcohol (aka No-Drink November). In this instance, you can cut the calories leading up to America's most overstuffed day of the year: Thanksgiving (and just days later, you'll be thankful for being able to drink in December as the holidays and parties roll around).

GIVE UP ALCOHOLIC LIQUIDS FOR LENT

Maybe you're religious, or maybe you've never been into organized faith. Either way, if you've given up on the no-beer journey, hop back on a couple months later. As many Christians do for Lent (the forty-day span before Easter), sacrifice a "luxury"—in this case: alcohol. Here's a chance to give up booze for even longer than any month on the calendar, if you so wish! Even if you're not Christian, participating in this tradition might bring you closer to your friends and family who are. You'll be able to be part of a community and share common ground with others who are also abstaining from a variety of things, including drinking.

SOBER OCTOBER

In case you weren't already tuned into this fall challenge (from reading all about it in this book, up until now): Nine months after Dry January ends, it's time for another thirty-one days without wine, beer, and spirits. Drumroll, please! Get ready for . . . Sober October! Like Dry Jan, Sober October is another (lesser practiced) nonimbibing challenge that eliminates all forms of booze—wine, beer, and spirits—for the entire month. Once summer has come and gone (along with the temptation and consumption of those fruity, light boozy beverages, including rosé and its cute slushy cousin frosé), and September has reacquainted everyone over happy hours with their long-lost friends and coworkers (long-lost, meaning August travel got in the way of seeing one another), October is time to buckle up for a French 75–free fall season.

The Chicago and DC marathons take place in October each year, and the New York marathon occurs the first weekend of November. If you're running any of these, best of luck to you (and remember to stretch)! But also, eliminating booze from your training schedule helps achieve better results. As previously mentioned: When you aren't imbibing, you're getting more restful sleep, which means your muscles and body will have a chance to relax and recover in between workouts. Alcohol also dehydrates the body, which isn't conducive to any form of cardiovascular exercise. Not a marathoner? No worries. You can still (not) drink like one!

When October 31 (Halloween) rolls around, instead of indulging in a drink (or a few), you can appropriately celebrate the near-end of your N.A. month with a sweet treat: candy! Chocoholics, taffy fanatics, and licorice lovers alike can reward themselves with a small (or large) gratifying snack. And even if you're not into gummies, lollipops, or other edible items, you can still dress up for the occasion (after all, it's another fun way to spend the day or night without imbibing)!

By the way, if you succeed during one dry month (like Dry January), you can absoluetly still crush another (like Sober October) later on in the year. (Consider it a zero-proof double shot.) Instead of eliminating booze for thirty-one days this year, overachievers unite! Really challenge yourself and go for the gold: sixty-two days without drinking (once in winter and once in fall). Of course, you're more than welcome to discard booze for longer than that back-to-back, or during nonconsecutive months, and any period of time in between! When it comes to limiting alcohol, you can go without it for as long as you'd like.

Don't Beat Yourself Up over It

If you've failed a dry month altogether, consider this a friendly intervention—but an encouraging one—with hugs and stuff! Don't get down on yourself or feel like a failure (at all!). Some people learn how to ride a bike on the first try (but not many). For most people, a bit of support (like training wheels) is needed. And even with help, things can still turn out badly (which is why helmets were invented). So, all in all, if you first fall down—literally, from drinking too much, or only in the figurative sense—just get back up again. The best thing you can do for yourself (and your Sober Month Support Squad) is keep trying. At the very least, even if you only manage to consume fewer drinks within the month, you've still made progress (and no bikes were harmed in the making of your dry month . . . hopefully).

A DAMP MONTH . . .

. . . that's a little less wet than Novembers in Seattle. If you've realized that a completely dry duration and a one-drink concession are out of the question (whether that's Day One, mid-month, or any time after), consider a damp month, e.g. Damp January. The notion isn't about throwing in the towel. It's an alternative to strictly abstaining from all

if you
fall down
just
get
back up
again

forms of alcohol (and giving yourself a bit more leeway). A Damp Month means you're consciously (and actually) making an effort to reduce your booze intake. Even if you haven't completely swiped your favorite bottle of Sauvignon Blanc from your diet, you're drinking far fewer glasses of it (and other boozy beverages) per month, compared to your regular routine.

There's Always Next Year

Peer pressure, celebrations, or a rough patch may have hijacked success, but just like trying out for the high school soccer team, if you don't make the cut this year, there's always next year, and other years to come.

Perhaps you didn't account for friends' and family celebrations every weekend of the month. Maybe your best friend had a baby the week before the scheduled due date (and celebrations were in order)!

Whatever the case, all is not lost.

You've likely changed some portion of your drinking habits during the month—or you've at least taken into account how your perspective around imbibing has shifted (even if it's minimal). You've still made progress. (So, go you!)

Even if you failed to reach your one and only New Year's goal, the best part of this less-than-ideal scenario is that the subsequent Dry January isn't light-years—or even a decade—away. Start again in eleven-ish months! By then, you'll be even more equipped and prepared to combat temptation. If you practice relaxing and dispelling stress in ways that don't involve drinking now, by next January you'll have personal, first-hand knowledge of how to replace imbibing activities with adventures that don't require bar crawls or body shots.

New Month's Eve

With one day left, you're almost at the finish line, trouper! Don't give up now. Even if you temporarily lost sight of your goals, go strong until the end and celebrate any (and every) large or small accomplishment you've made along the way!

In Case of Emergency

After declaring (and adopting) New Year's resolutions, it's easy to see why January, in general, is a month for revelations and growth. If, during your Dry January journey (or any other month), you find it's very difficult (like, really, really impossible) to forgo booze no matter what the situation—with friends, alone, in uncertain circumstances, or even familiar ones at all (or any random) hours of the day and night— and that your imbibing is perpetual (and in large quantities), please tell a friend, a family member, or a trusted individual. Realizing there's a potential problem can be both liberating and overwhelming. If you're having trouble carrying on with daily tasks, chores, and work without a drink, and you prefer to gain a little bit more information about your choices before divulging about your drinking regimen to people you know, please visit www.aa.org for more information and to find a phone number to the local Alcoholics Anonymous in your area. Another resource is the National Drug Helpline: drughelpline.org.

When Life Drops You Lemons, Do Not Reach for Vodka.
Repeat: Do Not Make a Lemon Drop

Good things (and change) take time! Looking for inspiration that proves you can, in fact, beat the odds? Hear from people who didn't give up during their pursuits to achieve some kind of greatness (likely not a month without booze, but that's beside the point!). These quotes may motivate you to come up with an empowering saying of your own!

"

Many of life's failures are people who did not realize how close they were to success when they gave up. —THOMAS A. EDISON

Your victory is right around the corner. Never give up. —NICKI MINAJ

Survival can be summed up in three words—never give up. That's the heart of it really. Just keep trying. —BEAR GRYLLS

I think a hero is an ordinary individual who finds the strength to persevere and endure in spite of overwhelming obstacles. —CHRISTOPHER REEVE

The successful warrior is the average man, with laser-like focus. —BRUCE LEE

The difference between successful people and really successful people is that really successful people say 'no' to almost everything. —WARREN BUFFETT

I'm disciplined And I'm persevering. And I don't give up very easily . . . and I'm reliable. —MADONNA

To succeed, we must first believe that we can. —NIKOS KAZANTZAKIS

The key to realizing a dream is to focus not on success but on significance—and then even the small steps and little victories along your path will take on greater meaning. —OPRAH WINFREY

If you don't go after what you want, you'll never have it. If you don't ask, the answer is always no. If you don't step forward, you're always in the same place. —NORA ROBERTS

"

To create your own personal dry month mantra, focus on what you truly desire and make your goals into a statement you want to stand by. Try jotting down a few ideas, then condensing those into a sentence, a phrase, or one or two words.

FOR EXAMPLE:
I want to feel in control, certain, and stable when I say no to drinking.
I am strong and certain.
Certainly strong.

You can have one or many mantras.

WRITE DOWN YOUR MOTIVATING MANTRAS, THOUGHTS, AND INSPIRATIONS HERE:

_____

_____

_____

_____

_____

_____

_____

_____

_____

Write your mantra on notecards and place them around the house or in one important spot, such as near your bed, so you can see those words of wisdom when you wake up in the morning and when you go to sleep at night. Take them to work, too. Make a note in your agenda book or a daily reminder in your phone calendar. Even tape them to the bottles of booze and wine that are still sitting on your bar cart or on top of your fridge (if you didn't ship off your stash or tuck it away)! Whip out these wise phrases when you're feeling as if you want a sip of wine, or to empower you when you're feeling strong, too.

CHAPTER 14

TGIF(inished)

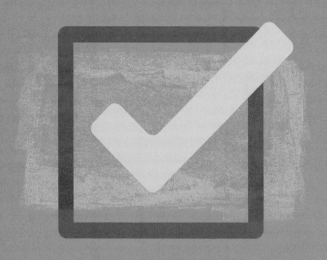

Thank goodness your dry month is finished! Congratulations, you made it to a new month—and without a sip of wine, beer, a mixed drink, or a teeny tiny shot glass of liquor. Following your month-long commitment to not drink a drop of alcohol, it's totally okay to enjoy a beverage (or two) in celebration (if you want to). You've not only survived, you've thrived—and you've earned a refreshing drink, after avoiding them for so long!

But before you jump back into your habits of yester-month (when you were someone who drinks socially, regularly, or very often), it's important to consider when, where, with whom, and how you should resurface into the world of imbibing. Whether you have a happy hour to attend or a full-blown party planned in honor of your reinitiation, there are a few elements to weigh prior to your first taste of alcohol.

Pace Yourself with That Piña Colada

If you've really missed wild, late nights out or chances to unwind at a bar after a long day at the office—and can't wait to mark your recent accomplishment—have the best time! (Really, no sarcasm.) But fair warning: It's very likely that your alcohol tolerance will not be the same as it was prechallenge (i.e., on December 31, for you Dry Jan'ers). Because science. And also, personal experience.

Case in point, titled "Don't Follow My Path If You Want to Wake Up the Next Morning Feeling Refreshed!"

Dry January Year One, February 1. I had two glasses of red wine. The result? A haze starting when I woke the following morning. My brain-fuzz continued until late afternoon. No amount of coffee or caffeinated tea could keep me from my fog. I felt as though I had consumed much, much more than two glasses of vino. . . . If my memory from December served me, it felt as though I had consumed four!

Year Two, February 1. The equivalent of two mixed drinks left me feeling down (specifically: sad and lethargic) the next day. Although past hangovers of yesteryear (during the thirty-one days prior) involved bouts of gloom, I had often associated it with the cold weather outside and the dark days! But, on this February 2, I realized it wasn't the sky—booze had depressed my mood.

Year Three, February 1. Just two vodka martinis had me craving unhealthy foods. (Yes, I actually purchased and consumed popcorn and ice cream that night . . . post-dinner. Hey, munchies happen, right?). Although I didn't give up my favorite snacks and treats during the previous thirty-one days, on the first night of February, I definitely consumed a larger serving of sugary goodies under the influence. Bloated and moving slowly for the rest of the weekend = not my best look.

Year Four, February 1. I didn't drink. I had no desire. My thirty-one-day dry challenge had concluded, and rather than commemorating it with a celebratory cocktail, I simply didn't consume (or want) any alcohol at all. By February 10, I had maintained my no-drinking streak and thought to myself, "Maybe I'll go on like this for another few weeks!"

You get the picture.

Acknowledging these potential results is key to not harming yourself (à la hangover) or others (by imposing your drunken idiocy on the masses). Take your time imbibing—and appreciating (rather than chugging)—each and every drink. Your friends might be eager to get you back out onto the party scene and generously offer to buy you copious amounts of shots, cocktails, beers, and more, but pace yourself (!!!!) and avoid gulping mouthfuls of single malts. Instead, swallow smaller portions slowly and with caution. Unless members of your Sober Month Support Squad (or other alcohol abstainers) are in attendance, the people you're boozing with won't be hit as hard as you are by the same quantity of beverages. (Spoiler alert: If you haven't taken the hint yet, your tolerance is likely 0.0, like that nonalcoholic beer you've been subbing in for your brewskis.)

pace
yourself
(!!!)

Beyond babysitting a beer, consider limiting yourself to one, two, or three libations for the night. Keep in mind: One size does *not* fit all. The number of drinks you can safely and comfortably consume depends on a number of factors: how long your outing is (one hour vs. twelve), how tall you are, how much you weigh, and also, what you've eaten or been drinking prior. (And, as a friendly reminder: The alcohol percentage per shots and cocktails vary. Same goes for wines and beers!)

In Preparation for Pints . . .

If enjoying a couple of cocktails is on the agenda for the day or evening, remember to eat something beforehand! Most drinkers can attest from personal, first-hand experience that consuming alcohol on an empty stomach is a surefire way to expedite intoxication (and inspire sickness later on . . . and the next day)! Food digested before or during drinking can slow the absorption of alcohol into the bloodstream. So whether you're vegan or a full-on carnivore: Eat!

And as you may have forgotten (due to lack of practice), it's also important to hydrate! Alcohol is a diuretic (meaning it dehydrates you at a more rapid pace). Therefore, pre-keg stand, pregame with water, and alternate boozy beverages with a glass of H_2O in between. (Your stomach and head will thank you later! Also, your friends will likely benefit from this as they won't have to help you walk straight or assist you in finding your way home. Or hold back your hair when that third marg rallies its way up to the surface.)

. . . and for the Aftermath of Absinthe

Plan for the future and stock up on your favorite antihangover foods for the hours and the morning after imbibing. Chugging H_2O before bed is ideal, but if that isn't your preference, try coconut water (which has a ton of potassium—more on this element in a minute)!

To save yourself from sickness, add more menu items, please. While it's important to consume food before and during your drinking excursions, it's also imperative to realize that not all dishes are created equal.

On the positive end of the spectrum: Eggs have amino acids that help boost liver function, and bananas contain potassium (alcohol's diuretic effect often depletes this mineral). In short: Breakfast is kind of your best friend. These morning-meal staples can save you from feeling your worst when the sun rises. On the negative side of the post-pisco food pyramid: Greasy foods are not so great for the day after drinking—so don't even think about ordering or cooking up a fatty meal! And, while you're at it, it's probably best that you avoid coffee (another diuretic), too—despite how much you need the caffeine!

"HAIR OF THE DOG"
If you're feeling hungover, do not consider drinking more booze! Not one drop! Contrary to popular belief, consuming more of what you had the night before will not cure a hangover. In fact, it can likely lead to even worse symptoms. (Gasp! As if you could feel *any* worse.) All in all, if you want to remedy nausea, stomach issues, and everything else that has been brought on by imbibing, opt for an N.A. beverage. (Side note: this will not undo any embarrassing moments you may have gotten yourself into the night before while intoxicated. Please consult your best friend or therapist for further instruction.)

SUPPLEMENTS TO STOP HEADACHES AND HANGOVERS (. . . OR SO THEY SAY)
In the wake of temporary alcohol-related illnesses, a plethora of antihangover remedies have made their way to market. (There are so many options that a big word like "plethora" was necessary.) Some of these products are preventive (so, you take them *before* imbibing), while others are palliative (an aftercare method that might serve you better than, say, oily hash browns). Taking the form of pills, tablets, powders, patches, liquids, and IVs, the promises to heal drink-related discomforts range in ingredients and price points. Not all are FDA approved, so read labels wisely and do your research to see what route is best for your needs. (Or consult your doctor for recommendations and feedback.)

Hitching a Ride Under the Influence

Regardless of your personality, be it an obsessive-compulsive planner or someone who does everything on the fly, it's imperative that you figure out how to get back home safely before you leave the house to celebrate your return to the bar. (Realistically, you haven't had to think about this for an entire month.) One option is to make sure a designated driver drops you off at the bar, and another suggestion is asking a friend or family member (who hasn't been drinking) to kindly pick you up (hi again, Mom!). In the instance where everyone wants to party, you can map out a route to your destination and utilize public transportation (if it's available in your area), virtually hire an on-demand car service, or hail a cab. If there are a number of people in your group planning to be under the influence, perhaps a party bus or limo is best to accommodate all guests—and their wallets. (But also: Who doesn't love a good car-hung disco ball with a soundtrack to match?)

Treat Yourself

Be honest: If you're human, it's more than likely that during the entire dry month, you've been promising yourself *something* to look forward to as you've been willing yourself to success. No judgment (or surprise) if you did! In fact, studies show that people will work hard to achieve goals when there are prizes at the finish line. If there's a will (read: a motivating shiny object that you really, really, really want at the end), then there's surely a way! If you've assured yourself there would be a margarita pitcher—or an equally oversized cocktail—waiting for you when you complete this challenge (in order to make it to the new month unscathed), then good for you! But please refer to page 209 about easing back into it . . .

Maybe keeping dry is working so well for you that you want to maintain your pact past your alotted month, or you prefer to celebrate without a beverage. In this case, reward yourself in a nonalcoholic fashion. (That's right, say "pass" to that solo or shared six-pack of beer. Also, go you!) Gifting yourself a massage or a fun workout class, taking yourself to a show, buying a new outfit, booking a trip, or finally checking out that hot new restaurant you've been dying to try (and have been endlessly stalking/salivating over on social media) are all satisfying ways to celebrate. (Hey there, truffle gnocchi—looking good!)

Perhaps the money you've saved, specifically from not drinking, can be the piggy bank for your (alcoholic or nonalcoholic) treat. And don't forget the bet winnings you've earned along the way!

CASHING IN ON YOUR BETS

Remember those high- (or low-) stake bets you made with friends before your challenge? While quickly filing through your notes or text messages, or simply revisiting chats from yester-month, you might be pleasantly surprised to find dinners, desserts, and other prizes await redemption—all thanks to your self-control! Not only did you save cash from not spending money on booze, but now your friends, family, and other bet-takers are going to treat you for sticking to your commitment! (What a deal!)

> **PRO TIP:** WHEN YOU GO TO COLLECT YOUR WINNINGS, SPREAD THEM OUT OVER THE COURSE OF A FEW WEEKS. IF YOUR BET CONSISTS OF A ROUND OF DRINKS, HAVING BACK-TO-BACK IMBIBING EXTRAVAGANZAS COULD BE MORE OF A CURSE THAN A GIFT.

Check, Please! (Your Goals, That Is)

When your challenge is over, you can continue to monitor how your life is shaped by the consumption—or elimination or reduction—of alcohol. The first day of the following month is a perfect time to reflect (and perhaps reread) your journal (or blog, video, calendar) entries and see how your mood, sleep, and social life (and piggy bank) changed over time—if at all. Specifically, revisit the notes you've scribbled on your worksheets within this book. Your day-to-day documentation is clear evidence of why you may feel or look better. You can certainly continue to jot down these details each day into the following weeks and months as you incorporate booze back into your diet. (Or don't—your choice!)

Touch base with your Sober Month Support Squad teammates—and all the other newfound and rekindled friendships you've built and strengthened since Day One. The new month is also a great time to reach out to amigos and other acquaintances you haven't been seeing much of (since you've spent a greater portion of time neglecting Negronis, and therefore avoiding late nights at the bar, and these individuals, too—only by coincidence, of course).

Bye-Bye Beer

While most dry month participants return to drinking alcoholic beverages after the month is complete, according to the *British Medical Journal* and Public Health England, up to 8 percent of the Dry January population are inspired to stay dry for a further five months. Perhaps you're not ready to commit to a six-month goal, in which case, you can certainly take it week by week or month by month! And research shows that even if you return to consuming cocktails, participation in a dry month leads to your drinking less even months later.

If you choose to continue forgoing all forms of alcohol, even once your challenge is over—whether it's another twenty-four hours of sobriety or an additional twenty-four months of declining beverages—good for you!

Do what makes you feel great, inspires happiness, and feels right.

Just like going dry for the entirety of January is best for some, the choice to pass on Pinot beyond the month is yours to make.

EXTENDING THE ELIMINATION OF ALCOHOL

If you were a Dry Jan'er and planning out thirty-one days of sobriety worked really well for you, try forgoing booze in February (it's a few days shorter)! Although the holidays and dates are different, the rules of no drinking apply just the same. And with the winter-season weather being relatively the same, most outdoor (and indoor) activities—that don't require drinking—are similar, and most important, just as fun!

Lessons Learned without Libations

After you've skimmed through your (paper or digital journal, voice memo, blog, or other reading material) entries, counted up your saved pennies, and/or evaluated how your body feels each morning, afternoon, and evening, you'll surely notice a difference—to one or more or all of these factors:

- an awareness of how eliminating alcohol impacts your day-to-day life: socially, in work settings, and physically;
- what there is to do around your town (besides drinking); and
- new skill sets you've adopted or taught yourself, like cooking, building things, and getting crafty.

As these special days—specifically carved out for an N.A. month—conclude, you'll likely realize you've learned a lot about yourself and other people around you.

The Last Drop (of Advice)

Regardless of how you celebrate the end of the month, it's important to recognize this is definitely a feat. Congratulate yourself on getting through all it!

For all of you who tried your best but didn't get all the way to your end date (Damp-Campers, that's you!), there's absolutely no reason to get down on yourself, either. You've still benefited from taking off even a couple of nights of imbibing. And, you've learned new, fun, productive, and entertaining ways to spend thirty-one consecutive days—without a drink in hand.

Finally, there is one major, unwavering fact about this trend that will surely never change, and it's the very best part about Dry January, Dry February, Dry July, Sober October, No-Drink November, or whatever dry month you choose:

If you want to do it better, differently, or challenge yourself again . . . there's always next year, or tomorrow!

Cong

rats...

. . . You've Made It!
(Now, Frame This.)

You've reached the end of your challenge, which can mean a few things as it pertains to not drinking! First and foremost, your dry stint is over. The start of a new month signifies your green light to become reacquainted with alcohol—a popular choice for most participants.

Going the distance should be commemorated (with or without booze)! Those who accomplished their goals (or at least did their best) should be proud.

In your honor, here is a certificate of achievement. Check off the one that suits your journey best!

CERTIFICATE OF
ACHIEVEMENT

This award is presented to

_____

[INSERT NAME HERE]

for participation in, and
[CIRCLE ONE]

- successfully consuming zero drinks during Dry January.
- minimizing alcohol intake during Damp January.
- observing Dry January and trying my best to eliminate alcohol.
- successfully consuming zero drinks during Dry/Sober

_____ .

[INSERT MONTH HERE]

- minimizing alcohol intake during Damp _____ .

[INSERT MONTH HERE]

- observing Dry/Sober _____ and trying my best
to eliminate alcohol. [INSERT MONTH HERE]

While doing so,

_____

[INSERT NAME HERE]

learned
[CIRCLE ONE OR MORE]

- how to socialize and have fun without booze.
- what it's like to turn down a cocktail and feel good about it.
- the ways abstaining from alcohol physically, financially, and mentally enhances day-to-day life!

_____   _____
HILARY SHEINBAUM   DATE
DRY JANUARY/SOBER MONTH EXPERT

Acknowledgments

Firstly, many thanks to my friend Alejandro. Without our bet, this book would have not been possible. You've inspired not only so many of my stories but also my terrible eating habits. (No, you cannot blame Tedy for this. Love you both.)

To my mother, who is still convinced there's time for me to go to law school so I can have a real career. (Mom: It's not happening. But thank you for your absurd persistence.)

For my father, who responds to my mother's wishes far more gracefully than I ever will. (You are a very, very special person. Also, thanks for not telling Mom about the incident—Mom, it's a joke.)

For Justin, Matthew, and Andrew: The number of memes that sum up our childhood is infinite. (Thanks for the laughs, and for two-thirds of you not being born on my birthday.)

For Leigh, who is the most badass City Cakes cookie-loving powerhouse. Thank you for always following up with me, answering literally seven thousand emails (mostly riddled with silly questions) and making things HAPPEN. Do you sleep? (Oh, and also major props for attempting Dry January. I'm convinced it will happen for you. Maybe next year. You have my number. Text me! Xoxo, Your Sober Month Support Squad.)

For Elizabeth, who has made my words more sensible and my sentences digestible. (I think I may have made up a word a few chapters back? I don't know for sure.) I'm so appreciative of your good vibes, positive attitude, and unlimited encouragement. And P.S., Hey, HarperCollins! I think you're pretty cool for taking a chance on a South Florida girl who's wanted to write a book since eighth grade (and thought giving up booze in January was a good idea). I'm forever thankful.

For my all editors, colleagues, fellow writers, and sources of the past and present (and all of the words cut from my copy and left behind). You have taught me so much about writing, editing, and life beyond my laptop. Also, shout-out to David (!!!!) for fixing said laptop (and my phone) . . . many, many times. P.S., to all: I'm sorry for temporarily hibernating while writing this book. On the bright side, it's done now.

And, for Will, who listens to all of my crazy ideas, enthusiastically supports (most of) my far-fetched editorial ideas, and gladly participates in my random challenges without hesitation (including Dry January). Thank you for all of it, and helping me get through many months of fun, silliness, and (sometimes) stress—with and without alcohol. (I think we have a few bridges to run in celebration . . . shall we?)

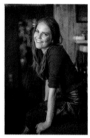

Hilary Sheinbaum has been a
Dry January participant and advocate since 2017.

As a reporter, she's covered topics ranging from celebrity red carpets to chef interviews, cocktail trends to new fitness classes, beauty treatments to wedding styles, and everything in between.

Her writing has appeared in the *New York Times*, *USA Today*, Today.com, *Travel + Leisure*, Yahoo!, and many other publications.

Hilary grew up in South Florida and attended both Florida State University (go Noles!) and the University of Florida (go Gators!). She currently resides in New York City.